Pediatric Colorectal Surgery

Pediatric Colorectal Surgery

Tips & Tricks

Marc A. Levitt, MD
Cheif, Division of Colorectal and Pelvic Reconstruction
Children's National Hospital
Professor of Surgery and Pediatrics
The George Washington University School of Medicine
Washington DC, USA

Associate Editors
Andrea Badillo, MD
Elise McKenna, MD, PhD
Rebecca Rentea, MD
Teresa Russell, MS

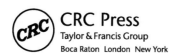

CRC Press
Taylor & Francis Group
Boca Raton London New York

CRC Press is an imprint of the
Taylor & Francis Group, an **informa** business

First edition published 2023
by CRC Press
6000 Broken Sound Parkway NW, Suite 300, Boca Raton, FL 33487-2742

and by CRC Press
4 Park Square, Milton Park, Abingdon, Oxon, OX14 4RN

Library of Congress Cataloging-in-Publication Data

Names: Levitt, Marc A. (Marc Aaron), 1967- author.
Title: Pediatric colorectal surgery : tips & tricks / by Marc A. Levitt.
Description: First edition. | Boca Raton, FL : CRC Press, 2022. | Includes
bibliographical references and index. | Summary: "Based on 30 years of
experience as a surgeon working in the field of pediatric colorectal and
pelvic reconstructive surgery, author Marc Levitt shares the tips and
tricks that he has developed to make operations and patient management
easier and reproducible. This book teaches these skills to achieve
positive results"-- Provided by publisher.
Identifiers: LCCN 2021062216 (print) | LCCN 2021062217 (ebook) | ISBN
9780367693176 (paperback) | ISBN 9780367712488 (hardback) | ISBN
9781003150015 (ebook)
Subjects: MESH: Digestive System Abnormalities--surgery | Infant, Newborn |
Child | Colorectal Surgery--methods | Rectal Diseases--surgery | Colonic
Diseases--surgery | Handbook
Classification: LCC RD543.C57 (print) | LCC RD543.C57 (ebook) | NLM WS 39
| DDC 617.5/547--dc23/eng/20220119
LC record available at https://lccn.loc.gov/2021062216
LC ebook record available at https://lccn.loc.gov/2021062217

ISBN: 9780367712488 (hbk)
ISBN: 9780367693176 (pbk)
ISBN: 9781003150015 (ebk)

DOI: 10.1201/9781003150015

Typeset in Minion
by Deanta Global Publishing Services, Chennai, India

CONTENTS

Part I: Anorectal and Cloacal Malformations

Part II: Hirschsprung Disease

Part III: Functional Constipation and Fecal Incontinence

Part IV: Post-PSARP and Post-HD Pull-Through Problems

Part V: Miscellaneous Colorectal Topics and Techniques

PREFACE

Patients with anorectal malformations (ARMs), Hirschsprung disease (HD), fecal incontinence from a variety of conditions, colonic motility disorders, and a myriad of other pathologies comprise the field of pediatric colorectal and pelvic reconstruction. Such patients require care from specialists across numerous fields throughout their lives, which may include colorectal surgery, urology, gynecology, and GI motility, as well as orthopedics, neurosurgery, anesthesia, pathology, radiology, psychology, social work, nutrition, and nursing.

Having met many parents with newborns diagnosed with colorectal problems, it is clear to me that no parent ever expects that their child would have a problem with stooling. This is a physiologic ability that is taken for granted, and when told their child has a problem with bowel function, they are usually hocked that something like this could ever occur. When discussing with these parents the necessity of surgery to correct their child's colorectal anatomy, none of them focus on the surgical technique and elegance of the anal reconstruction, which are the primary surgical goals. Parents are instead most concerned about whether the surgeon will create an anatomy that will allow their child to pass stool without difficulty and will keep them clean. As surgeons, it is our moral obligation to remember this. We always need to understand the result the family desires. As proud as we are of our surgical skills, it is the functional outcome that matters most to our patients and their parents.

In my 30 years of experience as a surgeon in this field working hard to improve the patients' quality of life, I have developed and learned from others a number of tricks that make operations or patient management easier. I talk about these often and teach them to trainees and colleagues. Many have asked me to write them down, and, in those requests, the idea for this book was born. I, together with the wonderful collaborators with whom I have worked on this book, have attempted to capture some of these special moments represented in the illustrated cases you are about to encounter. Our goal was to help other caregivers understand the daily struggle we experience in our work and to teach the readers of this book the skills and tricks to succeed.

Sometimes, the field of colorectal and pelvic reconstruction seems chaotic and unpredictable. Reconstruction requires creativity, and it may feel at times that artwork is being created during the actual operation, with no pre-plan in mind. I have worked very hard to counter that feeling, to be fully prepared, and to develop protocols and reproducible techniques and processes so that others can achieve optimal results for their patients. If, by doing this, I am able to help children I will never meet, then I will be very gratified.

Bringing order to chaos is well illustrated in an essay written by my daughter Jess, when she was a teenager, in which a series of somewhat random thoughts and ideas are, in fact, coordinated, once one understands the pattern that unifies them.

> *On the Alphabet*
> *"A" must come before "B," which must come before "C," everybody knows that. But what if the Millercamps of this world did not have to sit next to the Millerchips when it comes to seating arrangements? Can Pat Zawatsky be called before Jack Aaronson when the teacher is taking attendance? Do those 26 letters that make up all the dialogue, signs, thoughts, books, and titles in the English-speaking departments of the world need their specific spots in line? Everyone can sing you the well-known jingle from A to Z, but not many people can tell you why the alphabet is the way it is. For almost as long as humans have had language, they have had the alphabet.*
> *Good ole ABCs. However, the alphabet represents the human need for order and stability. I believe that the same thinking that went into the construct of time, and even*

government, went into the alphabet. Justifiably, lack of order leads to chaos. Knife-throwing, gun-shooting chaos, in the case of lack of governmental order. Listen to me when I tell you that there is absolutely no reason that the alphabet is arranged the way that it is. Moreover, the alphabet is simply a product of human nature and how it leads people to establish order for things that do not require it. Now I know this sounds crazy, but bear with me. Only if you really peel away the layers of the alphabet will you find the true weight it carries. People organized the letters of our speech into a specific order simply because there wasn't already one. Questioning this order will enlighten you on the true meaning of it. Really dig deep into the meaning behind the social construct that is the alphabet. Short and sweet as it may be, the order of the ABCs is much less than meets the eye. There is no reason that "J" should fall before "K!" Understand this. Very important as order is, it is only a result of human nature. What's next? X-rays become independent of Xylophones in children's books of ABCs? You know what the best part is? Zero chance you even noticed that each sentence in this essay is in alphabetical order.

I want to take this moment to thank my family, my wife, Shary, my children, Sam, Raquel, and Jess, my parents, Eva and Larry (Mom and Dad), my siblings, Adam and Lora, my acquired siblings, Sharone, Steph, Harly, and Becky, and my in-laws, Sandy and Abe, for your tireless support, devotion, and love. I would have achieved very little without you.

Marc A. Levitt, MD

EDITORS AND CONTRIBUTORS

ASSOCIATE EDITORS

- Andrea Badillo
  Director, Division of Colorectal and Pelvic Reconstruction and Attending Pediatric Surgeon
  Children's National Hospital, Washington DC, USA
- Elise McKenna
  Colorectal Fellow, Division of Colorectal and Pelvic Reconstruction
  Children's National Hospital, Washington DC, USA
- Rebecca Rentea
  Director, Comprehensive Colorectal Center
  Children's Mercy Hospital, Kansas, USA
- Teresa Russell
  Senior Clinical Research Coordinator, Divisions of Colorectal and Pelvic Reconstruction and Urology
  Children's National Hospital, Washington DC, USA

CONTRIBUTORS

- Hira Ahmad, Seattle, Washington, USA
- Alyssa Albany, Columbus, Ohio, USA
- Tamador Al-Shamaileh, Amman, Jordan
- June Amling, Washington DC, USA
- Anisha Apte, Washington DC, USA
- Yaron Armon, Jerusalem, Israel
- Krystal Artis, Washington DC, USA
- Jeff Avansino, Seattle, Washington, USA
- Christina Barnes, Columbus, Ohio, USA
- Rabab Barq, Richmond, Virginia
- Greg Bates, Columbus, Ohio, USA
- Elizaveta Bokova, Moscow, Russia
- Ivo deBlaauw, Nijmenen, Netherlands
- Kisha Bostic, Washington DC, USA
- Catherine Brennan, Cincinnati, Ohio, USA
- Giulia Brisighelli, Johannesburg, South Africa
- Dorothy Bulas, Washington DC, USA
- Margaret Cady, Washington DC, USA
- Kathryn Callicott, Washington DC, USA
- Susan Callicott, Washington DC, USA
- Kelci Campbell, Washington DC, USA
- Michelle Cantey, Washington DC, USA
- Cassie do Carmo, Columbus, Ohio, USA
- Lily Cheng, Houston, Texas, USA
- Julie Choueiki, Washington DC, USA
- Lindsay Clarke, Washington DC, USA
- Olivia Cleckley, Washington DC, USA
- Marissa Condon, Columbus, Ohio, USA
- Ted Copetas, Cincinnati, Ohio, USA
- Jackie Cronau, Columbus, Ohio, USA
- Anil Darbari, Washington, DC, USA
- Tazim Dowlut-McElroy, Washington DC, USA
- Sarah Driesbach, Columbus, Ohio, USA
- Allison Elsner, Cincinnati, Ohio, USA
- Tracey Farragut, Washington DC, USA
- Christina Feng, Washington DC, USA
- Kristi Ford, Washington DC, USA
- Katherine Forte, Washington DC, USA
- Chris Frake, Columbus, Ohio, USA
- Naftali Freud, Petach Tikvah, Israel
- Tarryn Gabler, Johannesburg, South Africa
- Katherine Gaddis, Salt Lake City, Utah, USA
- Justine Gagnon, Washington DC, USA
- Tara Garbarino, Washington DC, USA
- Keith Georgeson, Spokane, Washington, USA
- Veronica Gomez-Lobo, Washington DC, USA
- Miguel Guelfand, Santiago, Chile
- Kenia Hall, Washington DC, USA
- Devin Halleran, Portland, Oregon, USA
- Christina Ho, Washington DC, USA
- Dalia Hochstein, Washington DC, USA
- Kathleen Hoff, Atlanta, Georgia, USA
- Monica Holder, Cincinnati, Ohio, USA
- Stuart Hosie, Munich, Germany
- Shimon Jacobs, Washington DC, USA
- Marcus Jarboe, Ann Arbor, Michigan, USA
- Raj Kapur, Seattle, Washington, USA
- Patricia Kern, Cincinnati, Ohio, USA
- Andrea Kesar, Jerusalem, Israel
- Sundeep Keswani, Houston, Texas, USA
- Avery Kondik, Villa Hills, Kentucky, USA
- Jennifer Kondik, Cincinnati, Ohio, USA
- Steve Kraus, Houston, Texas, USA
- Martin Lacher, Leipzig, Germany

- Debra Lai, Washington DC, USA
- Victoria Lane, Newcastle, UK
- Jack Langer, Toronto, Canada
- Timothy Lee, Houston, Texas, USA
- Wendy Lee, Washington DC, USA
- Vickie Leonhardt, Columbus, Ohio, USA
- Celicia Little, Washington DC, USA
- Anna Marie Lukish, Washington DC, USA
- Eliana Maldonado, Washington DC, USA
- Connie Mantel, Seattle, Washington, USA
- Ivon Martinez, Washington DC, USA
- Allison Mayhew, Washington DC, USA
- Grace Ma, Washington DC, USA
- Michelle McGuire, Washington, DC, USA
- Mara Mercer, Washington DC, USA
- Meghan Mesa, Washington DC, USA
- Paola Midrio, Treviso, Italy
- Morgan Milner, Washington DC, USA
- Elizabeth Morrow, Washington DC, USA
- Susan Muma, Washington DC, USA
- John Myseros, Washington DC, USA
- Kurt Newman, Washington, DC, USA
- Jacqueline Newton, Washington DC, USA
- Vivien Pat, Washington DC, USA
- Allison Patton, Cincinnati, Ohio, USA
- Kathy Pazaropoulos, Columbus, Ohio, USA
- Lindsay Pesacreta, Washington DC, USA
- Tiffani Pietrucha, Washington DC, USA
- Hans Pohl, Washington DC, USA
- Kimberly Proos, Washington DC, USA
- Elena Puscasiu, Washington DC, USA
- Matt Ralls, Ann Arbor, Michigan, USA
- Carlos Reck, Vienna, Austria
- Emily Rice, Washington DC, USA
- LeTasia Robinson, Washington DC, USA
- Natalie Rose, Columbus, Ohio, USA
- Christopher Rossi, Washington DC, USA
- Eva Rubio, Washington, DC, USA
- Payam Saadai, Sacramento, California, USA
- Inbal Samuk, Petah Tikva, Israel
- Anthony Sandler, Washington DC, USA
- Sabine Sarnacki, Paris, France
- Nikki Scurlock, Washington, DC, USA
- Erin Shann, Columbus, Ohio, USA
- Karun Sharma, Washington, DC, USA
- Clare Skerritt, Bristol, UK
- Pim Sloots, Rotterdam, Netherlands
- Caitlin Smith, Seattle, Washington, USA
- Jennifer Stinebiser, Washington, DC, USA
- Jonathan Sutcliffe, Leeds, United Kingdom
- Laura Tiusaba, Washington DC, USA
- Thanos Tyraskis, Athens, Greece
- Rafi Udassin, Jerusalem, Israel
- Briony Varda, Washington DC, USA
- Karla Velasquez, Washington DC, USA
- Ranjith Vellody, Washington DC, USA
- Alejandra Vilanova Sanchez, Madrid, Spain
- Stephanie Vyrostek, Columbus, Ohio, USA
- David Wessel, Washington, DC, USA
- Chris Westgarth-Taylor, Johannesburg, South Africa
- Ginger Winder, Washington DC, USA
- Megan Wittenberg, Cincinnati, Ohio, USA
- Randi Wittenberg, Cincinnati, Ohio, USA
- Richard Wood, Columbus, Ohio, USA
- Katherine Worst, Washington DC, USA
- Bhupender Yadav, Washington DC, USA
- Jennifer Zeledon, Washington DC, USA
- Sarah Zobell, Salt Lake City, Utah, USA

FOR EVERYTHING A BLESSING

When I was an elementary school student in yeshiva – a Jewish parochial school with both religious and secular studies – my classmates and I used to find amusing a sign that was posted just outside the bathroom. It was an ancient Jewish blessing, commonly referred to as the *asher yatzar* benediction, that was supposed to be recited after one relieved oneself. For grade school children, there could be nothing more strange or ridiculous than to link acts of micturition and defecation with holy words that mentioned God's name. Blessings were reserved for prayers, for holy days, or for thanking God for food or for some act of deliverance, but surely not for a bodily function that evoked smirks and giggles.

It took me several decades to realize the wisdom that lay behind this blessing that was composed by Abayei, a fourth-century Babylonian rabbi.

Abayei's blessing is contained in the Talmud, an encyclopedic work of Jewish law and lore that was written over the first five centuries of the common era. The Jewish religion is chock-full of these blessings, or *brachot*, as they are called in Hebrew. In fact, an entire tractate of the Talmud, 128 pages in length, is devoted to *brachot*.

On page 120 (*Brachot* 60b) of the ancient text it is written:

> *Abayei said, when one comes out of a privy he should say: Blessed is He who has formed man in wisdom and created in him many orifices and many cavities. It is obvious and known before Your throne of glory that if one of them were to be ruptured or one of them blocked, it would be impossible for a man to survive and stand before You. Blessed are You that heals all flesh and does wonders.*

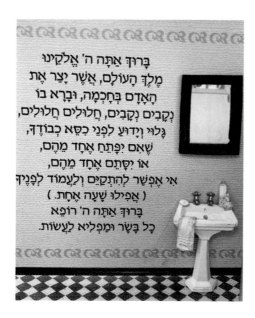

The *Asher Yatzar* prayer in Hebrew

An observant Jew is supposed to recite this blessing in Hebrew after each visit to the bathroom. We young yeshiva students were reminded of our obligation to recite this prayer by the signs that contained its text that were posted just outside the restroom doors.

It is one thing, however, to post these signs and it is quite another to realistically expect pre-adolescents to have the maturity to realize the wisdom of and need for reciting a 1600-year-old blessing related to bodily functions.

It was not until my second year of medical school that I first began to understand the appropriate-ness of this short prayer. Pathophysiology brought home to me the terrible consequences of even minor aberrations in the structure and function of the human body. At the very least, I began to no longer take for granted the normalcy of my trips to the bathroom. Instead, I started to realize how many things had to operate just right for these minor interruptions of my daily routine to run smoothly.

I thought of Abayei and his blessing. I recalled my days at yeshiva and remembered how silly that sign outside the bathroom had seemed. But after seeing patients whose lives revolved around their dialysis machines, and others with colostomies and urinary catheters, I realized how wise the rabbi had been.

And then it happened: I began to recite Abayei's *bracha*. At first, I had to go back to my *siddur*, the Jewish prayer book, to get the text right. With repetition – and there were many opportuni-ties for a novice to get to know this blessing well – I could recite it fluently and with sincerity and understanding.

Over the years, reciting the *asher yatzar* has become for me an opportunity to offer thanks not just for the proper functioning of my excretory organs, but for my overall good health. The text, after all, refers to catastrophic consequences of the rupture or obstruction of any bodily structure, not only those of the urinary or gastrointestinal tract. Could Abayei, for example, have foreseen that "blockage" of the "cavity," or lumen, of the coronary artery would lead to the commonest cause of death in industrialized countries some 16 centuries later?

I have often wondered if other people also yearn for some way to express gratitude for their good health. Physicians especially, who are exposed daily to the ravages that illness can wreak, must sometimes feel the need to express thanks for being well and thus well-being. Perhaps a generic, nondenominational *asher yatzar* could be composed for those who want to verbalize their grati-tude for being blessed with good health.

There was one unforgettable patient whose story reinforced the truth and beauty of the *asher yatzar* for me forever. Josh was a 20-year-old student who sustained an unstable fracture of his third and fourth cervical vertebrae in a motor vehicle crash. He nearly died from his injury and required emergency intubation and ventilatory support. He was initially totally quadriplegic but for weak flexion of his right biceps.

A long and difficult period of stabilization and rehabilitation followed. There were promising signs of neurological recovery over the first few months that came suddenly and unexpectedly: move-ment of a finger here, flexion of a toe there, return of sensation here, adduction of a muscle group there. With incredible courage, hard work, and an excellent physical therapist, Josh improved day by day. In time, and after what seemed like a miracle, he was able to walk slowly with a leg brace and a cane.

But Josh continued to require intermittent catheterization. I know only too well the problems and perils this young man would face for the rest of his life because of a neurogenic bladder. The urolo-gists were very pessimistic about his chances for not requiring catheterization. They had not seen this occur after a spinal cord injury of this severity.

Then the impossible happened. I was there the day Josh no longer required a urinary catheter. I thought of Abayei's *asher yatzar* prayer. Pointing out that I could not imagine a more meaningful scenario for its recitation, I suggested to Josh, who was also a yeshiva graduate, that he say the prayer. He agreed. As he recited the ancient *bracha*, tears welled in my eyes.

Josh is my son.

–Kenneth M. Prager, MD

ABOUT THE AUTHOR

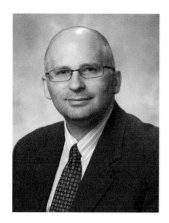

Marc A. Levitt, MD, has focused his career on enhancing the care of children with colorectal and pelvic reconstructive needs. He has cared for children from all 50 of the United States and over 75 countries and has performed more than 15,000 pediatric colorectal procedures. He has written three textbooks and this is his fourth, as well as over 300 scientific articles in this subject area. Dr. Levitt received his undergraduate degree from the University of Pennsylvania and his medical degree from the Albert Einstein College of Medicine. He completed his general surgery residency at Mount Sinai Medical Center, New York, a fellowship in Pediatric Colorectal Surgery at Schneider Children's Hospital, and a Pediatric Surgery fellowship at the Children's Hospital of Buffalo. His work extends to educating students, surgeons, other medical colleagues, and nurses, as well as developing integrated centers throughout the world to ensure that all children have access to quality colorectal care. He is actively engaged in helping patients, their doctors, and nurses in resource-limited locations through the organization Colorectal Team Overseas, www.ctoverseas.org. He is the Chief of the Division of Colorectal and Pelvic Reconstruction at Children's National Hospital in Washington DC, a uniquely integrated team of pediatric colorectal surgeons, urologists, gynecologists, gastroenterologists, advanced practice providers, and nurses, and is a Professor of Surgery and Pediatrics at The George Washington University School of Medicine.

PART I
ANORECTAL AND CLOACAL MALFORMATIONS

Chapter 1

NEWBORN ANORECTAL MALFORMATIONS

BABYLONIAN TALMUD

> I've learned that people will forget what you said, people will forget what you did, but people will never forget how you made them feel.
>
> **– Maya Angelou**

The Babylonian Talmud, an ancient and sacred text of the Jewish people written in the fourth century, is a compilation of the Mishnah, the oral law, and the Gemara, its rabbinical commentary. Tractate Shabbat, on page 134a, discusses the proper protocol for the situation in which a baby is born without an anus, or the hole for the exit of stool, which is covered by skin and is unable to be located. Abaye, a rabbi and a Jewish Talmud scholar in Babylonia, said 2000 years ago that, if these circumstances were to occur, one must rub the area with oil and have it be exposed to the sun. Then one should to take a grain of barley and tear the area widthwise and lengthwise, but should not use a metal instrument to make the tear because it can lead to infection and swelling. This may be the first reference to the modern-day surgical technique called an anoplasty (Figures 1.1 and 1.2).

Scanned Shas is ©Copyright Moznaim הוצאת ח. וגשל. Provided with their kind permission.

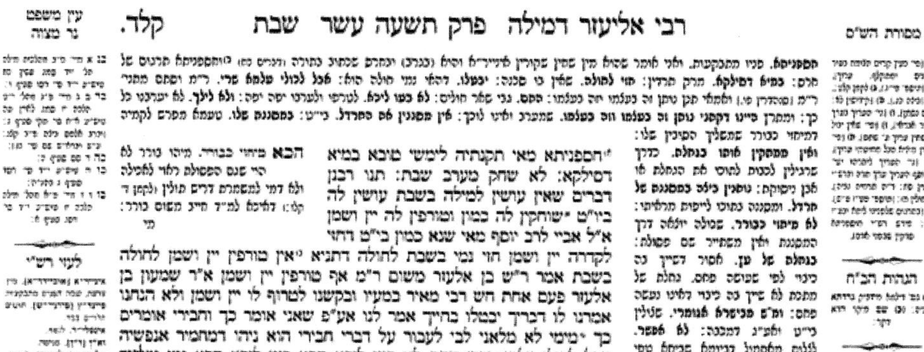

Figure 1.1 Ancient reference to treatment of an anorectal malformation.

DOI: 10.1201/9781003150015-2

Be curious, not judgmental.

– Contributed by: Marc Levitt

Babylonian Talmud: Tractate Shabbath

Folio 134a

What is his remedy? Let him wash it well in beet juice.

IF ONE DID NOT CRUSH [IT] ON THE EVE OF THE SABBATH. Our Rabbis taught: The things which may not be done for circumcision on the Sabbath may be done on Festivals: cummin may be crushed, and wine and oil may be beaten up together on its account. Abaye asked R. Joseph: Wherein does [the powdering of] cummin on Festivals differ? [presumably] because it can be used in a dish? then wine and oil too are fit for an invalid on the Sabbath? For it was taught: One may not beat up wine and oil for an invalid on the Sabbath. R. Simeon b. Eleazar said in R. Meir's name: One may indeed beat up wine and oil. R. Simeon b. Eleazar related, R. Meir was once suffering internally, and we wished to beat up wine and oil for him, but he would not permit us. Said we to him, Your words shall be made void in your own lifetime! Though I rule thus, he replied, yet my colleagues rule otherwise, [and] have never presumed to disregard the words of my colleagues. Now he was stringent in respect to himself, but for all others it is permitted? — There it need not be well beaten, whereas here it needs to be well beaten. Then let us do likewise here too and not mix it well? — That is what he teaches, EACH MUST BE PLACED SEPARATELY.

Our Rabbis taught: One may not strain mustard grain through its own strainer, nor sweeten it with a glowing coal. Abaye asked R. Joseph: Wherein does it differ from what we learnt: An egg may be passed through a mustard strainer? There it does not look like selecting, whereas here it looks like selecting, he replied. 'Nor sweeten it with a glowing coal'. But surely it was taught, One may sweeten it with a glowing coal? — There is no difficulty: one refers to a metal coal, the other to a wood coal. Abaye asked R. Joseph: Wherein does it differ from [roasting] meat on coals? — There it is impossible, whereas here it is possible. Abaye asked R. Joseph: What about cheese-making? — It is forbidden, answered he. Wherein does it differ from kneading [dough]? — There it is impossible, here it is possible, replied he. But the people of Nehardea say: Freshly-made cheese is palatable? — They mean this: even freshly-made cheese is palatable.

ONE MAY NOT MAKE A HALUK FOR IT, etc. Abaye said, Mother told me: The side-selvedge of an infant's haluk should be uppermost, lest a thread thereof stick and he [the infant] may become privily mutilated. Abaye's mother used to make a lining for half [the haluk].

Abaye said: If there is no haluk for an infant, a hemmed rag should be brought, and the hem tied round at the bottom and doubled over at the top.

Abaye also said: Mother told me, An infant whose anus is not visible should be rubbed with oil and stood in the sun, and where it shows transparent it should be torn crosswise with a barley grain, but not with a metal instrument, because that causes inflammation.

Figure 1.2 Ancient reference to treatment of an anorectal malformation.

NEWBORN COLOSTOMY

In an anorectal malformation (ARM, also known as imperforate anus), a divided colostomy is ideal, as it allows for egress of stool from the proximal segment and access to the distal segment to perform a distal colostogram. The stoma should be opened in the proximal sigmoid, leaving enough distal colon for the future pull-through. The proximal stoma is placed in the left lower quadrant, and the mucus fistula is made small and flat (Figure 1.3). A diverting loop colostomy is also a good option.

> Golf is a game of luck. The more I practice the luckier I get.
>
> – Ben Hogan

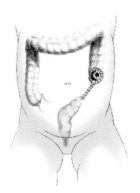 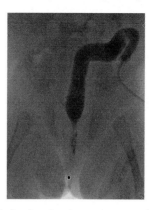

Figure 1.3 Stoma in the proximal sigmoid on the left, distal colostogram on the right.

The left photo in Figure 1.4 shows the traditional left lower quadrant oblique incision containing both stomas, with a skin bridge between the two stomas. The skin bridge can lead to skin troubles between the stomas. Because of the skin bridge issues, a laparoscopic approach can be used, whereby the two ends can be brought to different locations, with the mucous fistula made small and flat and the proximal stoma matured (shown in the right photo in Figure 1.4). This does make cleaning out the meconium more difficult, but it is still doable. Laparoscopy can be used to visualize the catheter placed into the distal segment during the irrigation process.

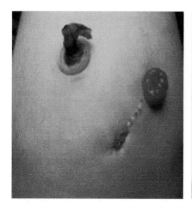 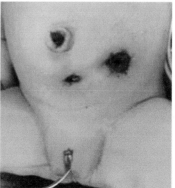

Figure 1.4 Traditional left lower quadrant stomas with a skin bridge between the two on the left, and no skin bridge on the right.

A Turnbull loop option with 95% of the proximal segment matured and the distal 5% left flat, creates a functional end stoma, but with access to the distal segment (Figure 1.5). This works very well and has several advantages: it is easy to create, the mesenteric vessels are not touched, and it is an easy stoma to close. The disadvantages are potential distal spillage of a loop (minimized by doing this Turnbull technique) and stomal prolapse. If your repair demands that there be no distal spillage, such as when the distal rectum has been redone, then an end stoma with or without access to the distal segment via a mucous fistula is a wise choice. Another nice trick is to pursestring close the mucous fistula to prevent spillage (Figure 1.6).

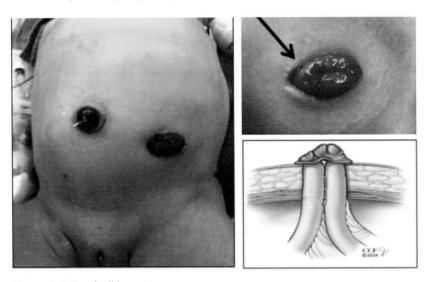

Figure 1.5 Turnbull loop stoma.

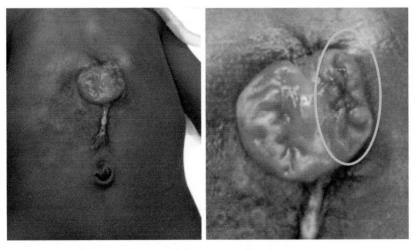

Figure 1.6 Pursestring closure of the mucous fistula.

RECOMMENDED READING

Liechty, ST, Barnhart, DC, Huber, JT, Zobell, S, Rollins, MD. The morbidity of a divided stoma compared to a loop colostomy in patients with anorectal malformation. *J Pediatr Surg.* 2016; 51(1): 107–110.

HOW TO EXAMINE THE FEMALE PERINEUM

Sometimes the female perineal examination is tricky, especially in newborns where all the structures are very small and close together. The external genitalia are also under maternal estrogen influence and may appear congested. It is helpful to examine the perineum from the front to the back, specifically noting the clitoris, labia,

> Alone we can do so little, together we can do so much.
>
> – Helen Keller

urethra, hymen, vagina, vestibule, perineal body, and anus. To observe the urethra and introitus, it is best to grasp the labia and pull them up and out. To observe the exact location of an anal opening, the perineal body should be pressed flat (Figure 1.7).

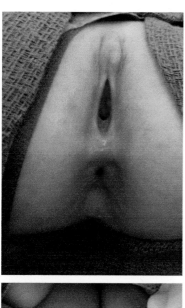

Check for:
- ✓ Clitoris
- ✓ Labia
- ✓ Urethra
- ✓ Hymen
- ✓ Vagina
- ✓ Vestibule
- ✓ Perineal Body
- ✓ Anus

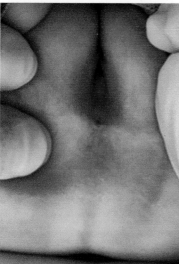
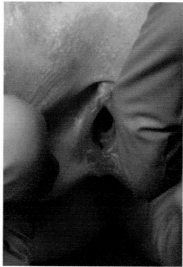

Figure 1.7 Examination of the female perineum.

FEMALE ARM VARIATIONS – SURGERY OR NO SURGERY?

Figure 1.8 shows photos of three different patients' perineums, with variations in the size and location of the anal orifice.

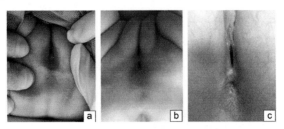

Figure 1.8 Three different females with ARM.

Do all these patients need surgery? If so, what technique would you use?

(a) This is a vestibular (almost Fourchette) fistula which needs the anal opening moved posteriorly into the center of the sphincter. Posterior or anterior sagittal anorectoplasty (PSARP or ASARP) and anal transposition (Potts) are all useful techniques. In all cases, it is vital to mobilize enough rectum so there is no tension on the anoplasty and to provide an adequately sized anus.

(b) This is a perineal fistula and also needs surgery.

(c) In this case, the physical exam alone is not enough, and the patient needs an exam under anesthesia with electrical stimulation. If the opening is adequately sized and there is some sphincter anteriorly, no surgery is needed.

The pictures in Figure 1.9 show the female perineal anatomy with the yellow dot representing the anal opening.

To summarize (from left to right in Figure 1.9):

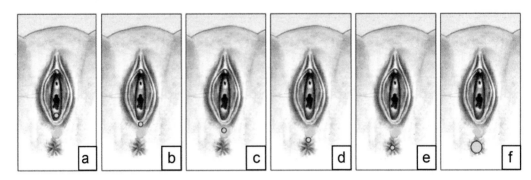

Figure 1.9 Female perineal possibilites.

(a) Vestibular fistula – needs surgery with rectal mobilization.

(b) Fourchette fistula – needs surgery with rectal wall mobilization.

(c) Perineal fistula outside the sphincter complex – needs surgery with rectal wall mobilization.

(d) Perineal fistula at the anterior extent of the sphincter complex – needs surgery with *only* posterior rectal wall mobilization.

(e) Normally positioned anus, but small size (anal stenosis) – needs anoplasty to make the anus normal size and screening for a presacral mass.

(f) Normal anus, but anteriorly located – no surgery needed.

ANORECTAL MALFORMATION IN A FEMALE NEWBORN – SURGERY OR NO SURGERY?

Let's test your knowledge: surgery or no surgery for the newborn female shown in Figure 1.10, with a normal urethra and normal vagina?

A good surgeon knows when NOT to cut.

– Contributed by: Sharon Cox

This patient has a very short perineal body with an anteriorly located anus. There is more pigmentation posteriorly, suggestive of the sphincter. However, the anal opening does appear to be within the sphincteric ellipse, just in the anterior portion. The anal opening appears otherwise normal. If it is the appropriate size, no surgery is needed for this patient. An examination under anesthesia (EUA) with electrostimulation to help determine the presence and size of the circumferential sphincter muscle would be very helpful.

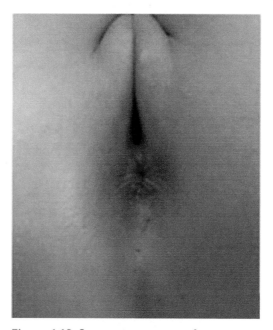

Figure 1.10 Surgery or no surgery?

An anus meeting the following criteria needs no surgical intervention:
1. Properly sized.
2. Surrounded by sphincter muscles.
3. An adequate perineal body.

In this case, all are true, and the anal canal also appears normal. The perineal body will grow over time. Moving this anus risks relocating it outside of the sphincter complex, leading to incontinence.

NEWBORN FEMALE WITH A PERINEAL ANOMALY

You see a newborn with a normal urethra, a normal vagina, and the anal anatomy shown in the photo in Figure 1.11.

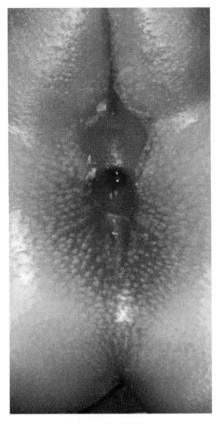

Figure 1.11 Female ARM.

Does she need surgery? If yes, what surgery would you offer?
This is a case of a perineal fistula with a perineal groove. The decision on surgery requires more information about the anus location and size first.

Is the anus the right size? Is it properly located within the sphincters?
If the hole is too small or is stenotic, then an anoplasty is needed. In this case, the anal opening appears to be too small and is located in the anterior-most portion of the sphincter (these facts can be confirmed with an EUA and electrostimulation). With an opening located in the anterior portion of the sphincter, you might only need to mobilize the posterior rectal wall. If the anus is not too small and not stenotic, it can be left alone, as the opening will function just like an anus, and being in the anterior-most portion of the sphincteric ellipse is of no clinical consequence.

Another key question is, if you had to intervene with an anoplasty to enlarge the anal opening, would you, at that point, do anything about the mucosa-lined perineal groove?
The answer is no – it will keratinize over time.

STIMULATION OF THE SPHINCTER COMPLEX

Identifying the muscle complex before and during a PSARP can be accomplished in an inexpensive and reproducible way. There are two options to perform muscle complex stimulation:

1. Attach a bipolar diathermy handle to the nerve stimulator (see Figure 1.12). Use the open ends of the diathermy handle on a well-lubricated perineum (be sure not to close the ends while stimulating as this could cause burns to the skin).

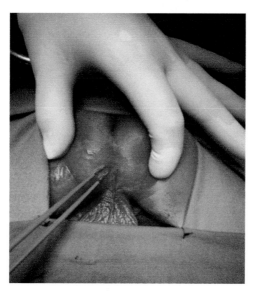

Figure 1.12 Bipolar diathermy used as electrical stimulator.

2. Attach two needles to the stimulator (see Figure 1.13). The stimulator can be placed in a sterile bag, and the probes connected through the plastic.

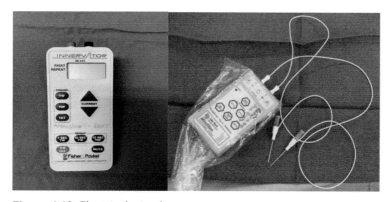

Figure 1.13 Electrical stimulator.

RECOMMENDED READING

Kapuller, V, Arbell, D, Udassin, R, Armon, Y. A new job for an old device: a novel use for nerve stimulators in anorectal malformations. *J Pediator Sung.* 2014 Mar; 49(3): 495–496.

CHAPTER 2

PREDICTORS OF CONTINENCE

IMPORTANCE OF THE SACRAL RATIO IN PREDICTING BOWEL CONTROL

A 4-year-old male with a history of ARM presents to the clinic. The patient had a rectoprostatic fistula that was repaired and a spinal cord de-tethering. Figure 2.1 shows his sacral films.

If every eight year old in the world is taught meditation, we will eliminate violence from the world within one generation.

– 14th Dalai Lama

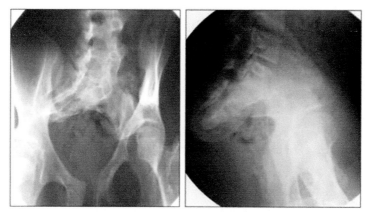

Figure 2.1 AP and lateral views of the patient's sacrum.

1. Can you calculate the sacral ratio (BC/AB) in AP and lateral projections?

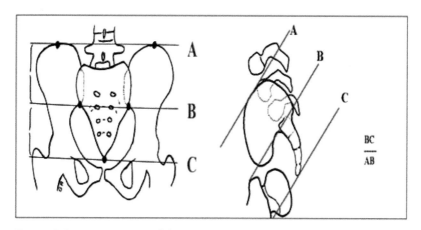

Figure 2.2 Measurement of the sacral ratio.

DOI: 10.1201/9781003150015-3

2. What does this assessment of the sacrum mean regarding the patient's prognosis for bowel control, i.e. does it help in the conversation with the family about their child's ability to achieve voluntary bowel movements?

If you respect tissue, tissue will respect you.

– Contributed by: Rambha Rai

The sacrum is a good indicator of the development of the pelvis. If the sacrum has formed well, it is likely that so too have the surrounding muscles and nerves. ARM patients have varying degrees of associated sacral hypodevelopment. What is important to notice in this case is that, in the AP view, it appears as if no sacrum is present; however, the lateral view demonstrates a reasonably good sacrum (Figure 2.1). The difference is because the tilt of the pelvis can give a falsely low sacral ratio in the AP projection. The AP view of the sacrum is really only used to check for a hemisacrum. The lateral image is needed for accurate sacral ratio calculation (Figure 2.2).

The sacral ratio is calculated on the lateral X-ray as demonstrated in Figure 2.3.

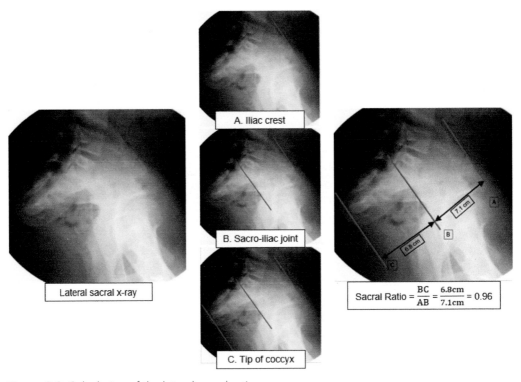

A. Iliac crest

B. Sacro-iliac joint

C. Tip of coccyx

Lateral sacral x-ray

$$\text{Sacral Ratio} = \frac{BC}{AB} = \frac{6.8\text{cm}}{7.1\text{cm}} = 0.96$$

Figure 2.3 Calculation of the lateral sacral ratio.

PREDICTING CONTINENCE IN AN ANORECTAL MALFORMATION PATIENT

Clinicians caring for an ARM patient should always know the type of malformation, the quality of the spine, and the quality of the sacrum. With those three elements, they can have a good idea of the patient's potential for bowel control. The chart in Figure 2.4 is a helpful guide to discuss this issue with patients. Even with the ARM Continence Predictor Index, predictions for some cases will remain uncertain. For example, for a patient with a rectoprostatic fistula, an intermediate sacrum, and a tethered cord, the prognosis is hard to predict.

The plural of anecdote is not data.

– Fred Ryckman

In this life, we cannot do great things. We can only do small things with great love.

– Mother Teresa, Contributed by: Teresa Russell

ARM Continence Predictor Index

		Number
ARM TYPE	Perineal Fistula	1
	Anal Stenosis	1
	Rectal Atresia	1
	Rectovestibular Fistula	1
	Rectobulbar Fistula	1
	ARM without Fistula	1
	Cloaca<3 cm Common Channel	2
	Rectoprostatic Fistula	2
	Rectovaginal Fistula	2
	Rectobladderneck Fistula	3
	Cloaca>3 cm Common Channel	3
	Cloacal Exstrophy	3

		Number
SPINE	Normal termination of the conus (L1-L2)	1
	Normal filum appearance	1
	Abnormally low termination of the conus (below L3)	2
	Abnormal fatty thickening of filum	2
	Myelomeningocele	3

		Number
SACRUM	Sacral Ratio equal to or greater than 0.7	1
	Sacral Ratio less than 0.69 or greater than 0.4	2
	Hemisacrum	2
	Sacral hemivertebrae	2
	Presacral mass	2
	Sacral Ratio less than 0.4	3

TOTAL NUMBER

3-4 = Good Potential for Continence

5-6 = Fair Potential for Continence

7-9 = Poor Potential for Continence

Figure 2.4 ARM Continence Predictor Index.

These elements and their respective weights need to be validated across hundreds of patients, a project currently being undertaken by the Pediatric Colorectal and Pelvic Learning Consortium (www.pcplc.org) to know each element's exact contribution to continence. For now, they are a useful aid in conversations about prognosis with families.

The surgeon should start by evaluating the patient's potential for bowel control using the ARM Continence Predictor Index (Figure 2.4). This index consists of three parts: the type of ARM, the sacral ratio (SR; calculated from the lateral view of the sacrum), and the quality of the spine (seen on spinal MRI), each assigned a numerical values. The values are summed to calculate a number, which will inform the conversation regarding a poor, fair, or good potential for bowel continence.

CHAPTER 3

OPERATIVE DECISION MAKING

HOW BEST TO FIND THE RECTUM? VIA A POSTERIOR SAGITTAL OR A LAPAROSCOPIC APPROACH?

Sometimes, it is not easy to determine whether to do a PSARP-only approach or a PSARP with laparoscopy (also known as laparoscopic-assisted anorectoplasty, LAARP). To help decide, draw a horizontal line starting at the tip of the coccyx to the pubic bone.

> Every decision should be based on the 'What if it were my child?' paradigm.
>
> **– Contributed by: Megan Durham**

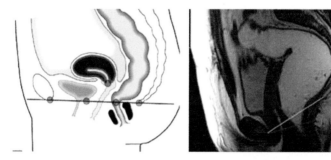

Figure 3.1 To determine whether to do a PSARP only or a PSARP with laparascopy, use the PC line.

This line is the pubo-coccygeal (PC) line, also affectionately known as the "Alejandra line", where the pelvic muscles normally compress the rectum. If, via a posterior sagittal approach, the first structure encountered below the PC line would be the rectum (Figure 3.2a), then a PSARP is best. However, if the first structure encountered below the PC line would be the urogenital anatomy (Figure 3.2b), then laparoscopy or laparotomy is needed to best identify the rectum and avoid injury to the or gynecologic urologic systems.

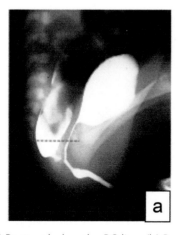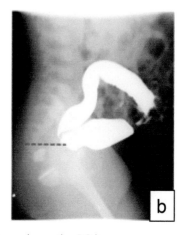

Figure 3.2 (a) Rectum below the PC line, (b) Rectum above the PC line.

LAPAROSCOPIC-ASSISTED VS POSTERIOR SAGITTAL ANORECTOPLASTY

The position of the rectum in relation to the PC line helps the surgeon determine the optimal surgical approach of PSARP or LAARP. A well-performed high-pressure distal colostogram can help predict the optimal surgical approach based on the presence of the rectum above or below the PC line.

Selecting a laparoscopic approach for a rectum that is below the peritoneal reflection may result in unnecessary intra-abdominal mobilization (leading to prolapse and ischemia) of the rectum and risks leaving a remnant of the original fistula (ROOF) on the urethra, which may require reoperation.

Figure 3.3 shows a magnetic resonance image (MRI) of the pelvis demonstrating a multilobulated mass which was the ROOF (short arrow) in a patient following a laparoscopic ARM operation which was done for a rectobulbar urethral fistula. There is a catheter in the rectum (long arrow). Because the approach to this low rectum was from above, the surgeon never reached the distal rectum, and inadvertently left it behind. The ROOF can lead to urinary tract infections (UTIs), mucous in the urine, stone formation, and potentially cancer development in the colon remnant bathed by urine.

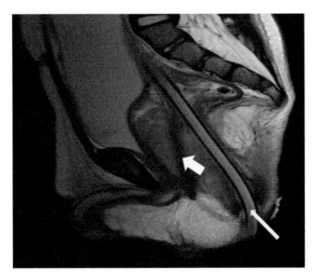

Figure 3.3

RECOMMENDED READING

Rentea RM, Halleran DR, Vilanova-Sanchez A, Lane VA, Reck CA, Weaver L, Booth K, DaJusta D, Ching C, Fuchs ME, Jayanthi RR, Levitt MA, Wood RJ. Diagnosis and management of a remnant of the original fistula (ROOF) in males following surgery for anorectal malformations. *J Pediatr Surg.* 2019 Oct; 54(10): 1988–1992.

A RARE TYPE OF PERINEAL FISTULA

A 6-month-old male infant with ARM, who underwent a colostomy as a newborn, presents to your clinic. A distal colostogram is demonstrated in Figure 3.4.

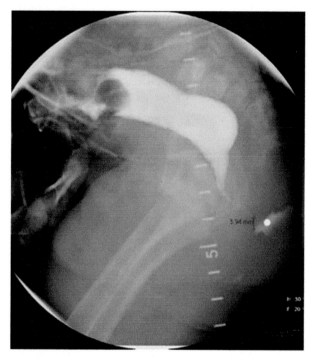

Figure 3.4

How would you describe this malformation?

This is a rare case of a long, narrow perineal fistula. This case is rare because most patients with perineal fistulae have a normal caliber rectum starting within 1–2 cm proximal to the fistulous tract to the perineal skin. In this case, the fistula is long and narrow, and the healthy rectal lumen is higher than the coccyx. Recognize that the distal rectum is compressed at the PC line, so there is more rectum distally than what is seen on the contrast study, because the rectum is not fully distended as the contrast flows out of the fistula.

> You can't improve on an asymptomatic patient.
>
> **– Siggie Ein, Contributed by:**
> **Jack Langer**

What repair would you choose?

The distal rectum in this case is reachable via a posterior sagittal approach. In most perineal fistulae, the surgeon would approach such a patient in the newborn period and can expect to find the rectum close by. However, in the rare situation shown in this case, the surgeon could have realized the rectum was too high during the dissection and instead chosen to perform a colostomy and then plan a future repair.

WHERE IS THE RECTOURINARY FISTULA?

The concept to help delineate the types of rectourethral fistulae in a male with ARM was inspired when this book's author saw the sculpture of Saint John the Baptist by Auguste Rodin at the Musée d'Orsay in Paris. When doing a distal colostogram to identify the type of fistula, the anatomy can be compared with the arm of this statue, which is used in Figure 3.5 to illustrate the course of the male urethra. The elbow represents the bulbar urethra, the humerus represents the prostatic urethra, and the axilla represents the bladder neck. Using this construct, clinicians can be consistent in the description of the distal rectal anatomy.

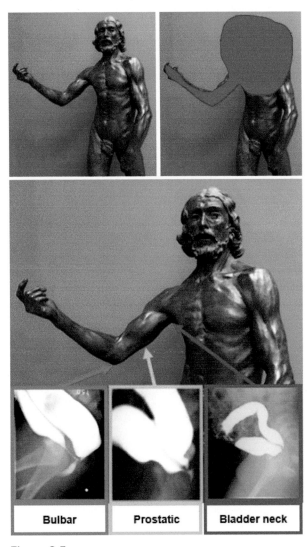

Figure 3.5

RECOMMENDED READING

Halleran DR, Ahmad H, Bates DG, Vilanova-Sanchez A, Wood RJ, Levitt MA. A call to ARMs: Accurate identification of the anatomy of the rectourethral fistula in anorectal malformations. *J Pediatr Surg*. 2019 Aug; 54(8): 1708–1710.

ANORECTAL MALFORMATION WITH A VERY LOW BULBAR FISTULA

A newborn, diagnosed shortly after birth with ARM, has a perineal exam and a cross table lateral film (done at 24 hours), which are shown in Figures 3.6 and 3.7. The patient has no evidence of meconium on the perineum or in the urine.

> Everything in moderation, including moderation.
>
> **– Oscar Wilde**

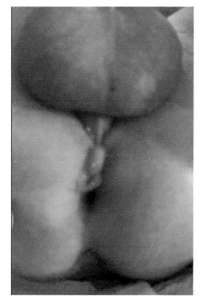

Figure 3.6 Perineal exam

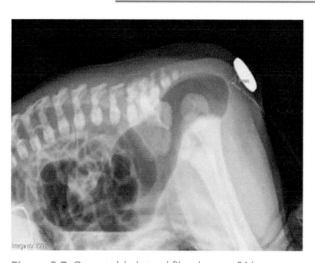

Figure 3.7 Cross table lateral film done at 24 hours

How would you approach this patient?

Looking at the X-ray, you can see that this patient has a very low rectum. Most likely this is a low rectum with no fistula or a rectoperineal fistula not yet visible on the skin. However, there is a possibility that this patient has a urethral fistula. A repair done in the newborn period might have led to a key pitfall – doing an anoplasty and not realizing there was a urethral fistula. Later, the patient would start to pass urine via the anus and would require a complete redo.

Would you do a primary anoplasty or a colostomy?

A colostomy would be the safest move. It allows you to do a colostogram and identify the fistula before surgery. However, if you approach this patient using a primary repair and understand that there is the possibility of a rectobulbar fistula, then a repair can be done safely in the newborn period. Such a repair should include the opening of the posterior rectal wall, careful inspection of the anterior rectal wall, and then mobilization of the rectum off the urethra with the repair of the rectobulbar fistula if one is found.

ANORECTAL MALFORMATION WITH NO FISTULA

You see a male patient with an ARM. The patient underwent a voiding cystourethrogram (VCUG) and a distal colostogram, the results of which are shown in Figure 3.8.

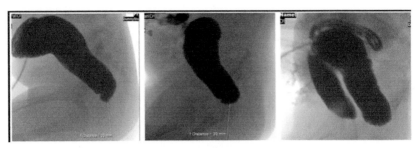

Figure 3.8

What malformation does the patient have?

Because the distal colostogram demonstrates a rounded distal rectum, this patient appears to have an ARM without a fistula defect. The contrast in the bladder can be explained by the fact that the colostogram and the VCUG were performed at the same time.

Which surgery would you perform (a PSARP or a laparoscopic procedure)?

The rectum is reachable via a posterior sagittal incision as the distal rectum is below the PC line (Figure 3.9). Laparoscopy could also be a useful approach, as this abnormality is higher than the typical no fistula defect (which usually is at the same level as a rectobulbar fistula). Remember that the no-fistula defect is often associated with Down syndrome.

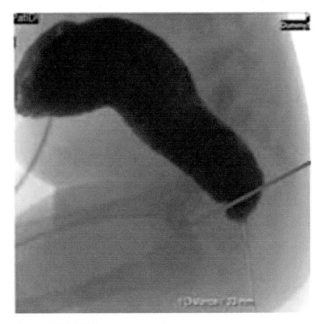

Figure 3.9 PC line is shown in blue.

ANORECTAL MALFORMATION WITH THE RECTAL FISTULA IN THE SCROTAL RAPHE

A full-term newborn with ARM has no anal opening and meconium was noticed passing through a fistula in the scrotal raphe.

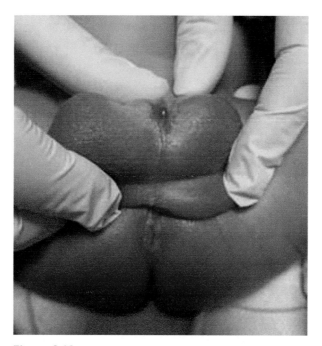

Figure 3.10

How would you manage this patient? Would you do a colostomy or a primary repair?

In Figure 3.10, you can see an anal dimple at the sphincteric ellipse. The opening in the scrotal raphe could be hypospadias, urethral duplication, or a rectoperineal fistula.

In this patient, it is a perineal fistula, as meconium is visible and there is no anal opening. Therefore, in this case, the good rectum can be expected to be very close – within 1 cm – of the location of the desired anoplasty. However, the fistula is long and runs right along the urethra. A primary repair is possible but will be difficult and carries the risk of urethral injury. A colostomy is a very safe option in this case. At the main repair, the fistula does not need to be dissected out, just the subepithelial raphe unroofed. This will avoid injury to the urethra.

Hard work always beats intelligence.

– Contributed by: Naeem Liaqat

HIGH RECTUM WITH NO FISTULA OR INADEQUATE CONTRAST STUDY?

A newborn male with an ARM underwent a colostomy. A few days later, a bead of meconium appeared at the upper scrotal raphe at the base of the penile shaft. The distal colostogram can be seen in Figure 3.11.

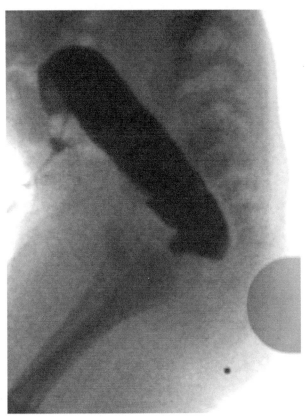

Figure 3.11

What is the anorectal diagnosis?

The surgeons who managed this case began with laparoscopy because of a misread of this colostogram. They found during their dissection that the rectum in fact went below the peritoneal reflection. An intraoperative colostogram confirmed a very low rectum, and the anoplasty was completed from a posterior sagittal approach. The radiologic study shown in Figure 3.11 did not provide adequate pressure and should have been repeated preoperatively. The flat line on the image should have been recognized as normal compression of the rectum by the pelvic inlet muscles. This line corresponds to the PC line. Therefore, the imaging is falsely showing a "high" rectum, but, as evidenced by the meconium appearing at the scrotum, the rectum is actually very low.

What would you do?

For a very low rectum, a posterior sagittal approach is preferable. You should not dissect out the fistula which heads anteriorly toward the scrotum and parallels the urethra. It will disappear over time after you have mobilized the distal rectum, making sure the anterior rectum is nicely separated and mobilized for the anoplasty. Chasing the fistula would be dangerous because of the risk of spongiosum bleeding and urethral injury.

POSTERIOR SAGITTAL ANORECTOPLASTY OR LAPAROSCOPY?

A child with an ARM has the distal colostogram shown in Figure 3.12.

Forgive others, not because they deserve forgiveness, but because you deserve peace.

– Jonathan Lockwood Hule

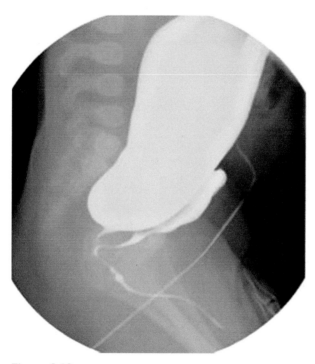

Figure 3.12

Which approach would you choose: PSARP or laparoscopy?

In this challenging case, the rectum is very high, above the PC line. The rectum is also quite bulbous. The height of the rectum makes laparoscopy an easier approach. In this rare case, although the rectum is high, the fistula is at the bulbar level, right at the elbow of our earlier referenced sculpture (Figure 3.5). The distal rectal dissection will be challenging because the rectum is so wide.

In a posterior sagittal approach, the surgeon would need to look way above the coccyx to find the rectum. If you do not have this clear image in advance, a posterior sagittal approach risks injury to the urinary tract.

POSTERIOR SAGITTAL ANORECTOPLASTY OR LAPAROSCOPY?

A high-pressure distal colostogram in an ARM patient is shown in Figure 3.13.

Judging a person does not define who they are. It defines who you are.

– Amy Rees

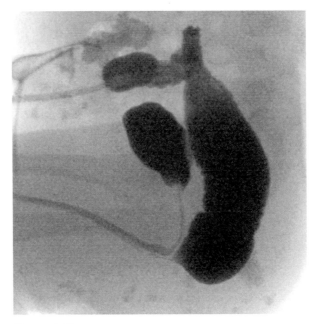

Figure 3.13

What is unique about the rectourethral fistula?

This is a case of a low rectobulbar fistula, and what is particularly noteworthy is the long thin fistula that parallels the urethra.

Which approach would you choose: laparoscopy or PSARP?

A PSARP is the best approach in this case. The fistula to the urethra needs a few sutures, and the anterior rectal wall needs to be fully mobilized. The long thin part of the fistula should be left alone (without any dissection). It will disappear and be of no consequence. Similar to the previous case with the fistula in the scrotal raphe, dissecting out the fistula puts the patient at risk for a urethral injury and significant periurethral spongiosum bleeding.

CHAPTER 4

OPERATIVE TECHNIQUES

LIGATING A RECTOBLADDERNECK FISTULA LAPAROSCOPICALLY

For a patient with a rectobladderneck fistula, dissection of the distal rectum down to the bladder neck is key. Once adequate dissection has been performed, a PDS Endoloop™ is inserted into the abdomen. To prepare for division of the fistula, a 3 mm Maryland instrument can be utilized to grasp the fistula after passing it through the Endoloop™. The Maryland clamp closes the fistula. The

A kutya ugat, esh a caravan halad. The dogs bark but the caravan moves on. (Translated from Hungarian)

– Contributed by: Olga Ritter and Marc Levitt

fistula is then divided (while maintaining control of the fistula with the Maryland clamp) utilizing laparoscopic scissors. The Endoloop™ is then brought over the Maryland grasper to ligate the fistula (Figure 4.1).

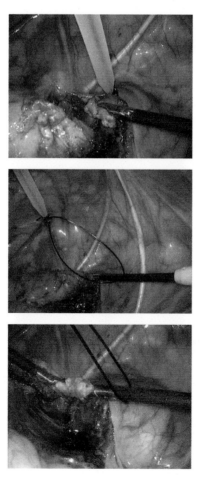

Figure 4.1 Ligating a rectobladderneck fistula laparascopically.

DOI: 10.1201/9781003150015-5

RECTAL DISSECTION

It's not the unanswered questions that matter most but rather the unquestioned answers.

– Alberto Peña

During a PSARP for ARM or a transanal pull-through for HD, it can be challenging to find the vitally important plane that will allow the rectum to be adequately mobilized to reach the perineum. One trick is to identify the shiny layer of fat. If you can identify that shiny layer of fat, you will know that you still need to get closer to the rectum with your dissection (Figure 4.2). If you see fat, you can get closer.

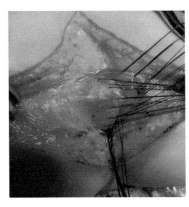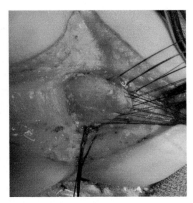

Figure 4.2 Whitish plane that encapsulaters the rectum.

And remember the famous words of Tattoo from the TV show *Fantasy Island* and be happy when you have found "Da plane, da plane" (Figure 4.3).

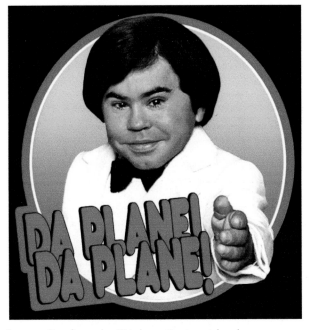

Figure 4.3 Tattoo's famous line from the TV show *Fantasy Island*.

PSARP EXPOSURE

To gain proper exposure during a PSARP dissection, it is helpful to use a combination of retraction with a Weitlaner self-retaining retractor and lone star pins. Placing a lone star pin at the 12 o'clock position is particularly helpful, especially if the rectum is high (Figure 4.4).

Stupid people don't know they are stupid, because they are stupid.

– Contributed by:
Vadim Kapuller

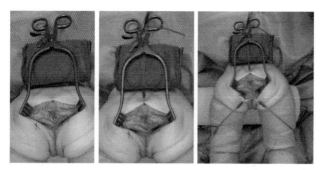

Figure 4.4 Weitlaner self-retaining retractor plus lone star pins provide excellent exposure.

HOW TO GET A HIGH RECTUM TO REACH – DISSECTION OF THE VESSELS

Getting a high rectum to reach the perineum for the repair of a rectobladderneck fistula is a considerable challenge. There are two important tricks for mobilization of the rectum that can be used. The first is the dissection of the vessels and the second is tapering of the bowel using a Heineke–Mikulicz (HM) rectoplasty.

Dissection adjacent to the rectal wall allows the surgeon to gain length on the rectum while preserving the IMA branch, which provides the intramural blood supply to the rectum. This dissection is illustrated in Figure 4.5.

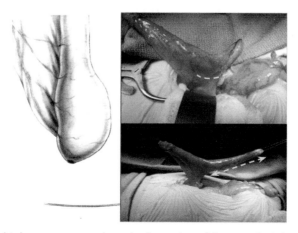

Figure 4.5 Getting a high rectum to reach — via dissection of the vessels right next to the rectal wall.

HOW TO GET A HIGH RECTUM TO REACH – TAPERING THE BOWEL: HEINEKE–MIKULICZ RECTOPLASTY

Fortune favors the prepared mind.

— **Louis Pasteur**

Sometimes, in a male patient with an ARM involving a rectobladderneck fistula, the distal rectum is very high, far away from the perineum, and bulbous in appearance. These factors set up a situation whereby an HM rectoplasty of the antimesenteric bowel can be very helpful. An incision is made transversely across the bowel and closed longitudinally. The maneuver will gain approximately 2–3 cm and will also taper the bowel's dilated distal end (Figure 4.6).

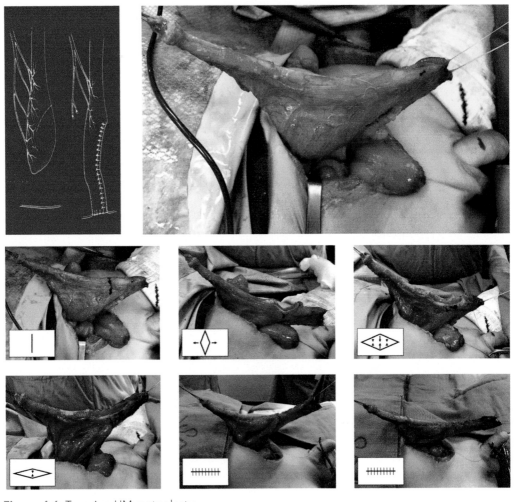

Figure 4.6 Tapering HM rectoplasty.

THE PERINEAL INCISION FOR A LAPAROSCOPIC–ASSISTED ANORECTOPLASTY

For an ARM patient with a high rectoprostatic or a rectobladderneck fistula, the operation for the pull-through begins in the abdomen with a laparoscopic dissection (or via laparotomy) of the distal rectum and ligation of the fistula. Once the rectum has enough mobility, it is time for the rectum to be brought through the pelvis to the perineum. It is important to preserve the blood supply of the rectum, which depends on the IMA and its branches on the rectal wall, which provide intramural blood supply. A small perineal incision is made. Then, using a mosquito clamp, the surgeon dissects just in front of the coccyx and sacrum and passes the clamp into the peritoneum (under laparoscopic visualization), staying clear of the urethra and bladder. Finger dissection between the pubic bone and sacrum to make the space is very helpful. This dissected space is now visible laparoscopically and the rectum is grasped and pulled through, maintaining a normal rectal angle and taking great care not to twist the pull-through. The direct perineal visualization of the sphincter complex through confirmatory electrical stimulation, midline dissection, and dilation is preferred to the blind placement of a large trocar. In addition, the small posterior sagittal incision allows for tacking of the posterior rectal wall to the muscle complex, as with a standard PSARP, to prevent rectal prolapse (Figure 4.7).

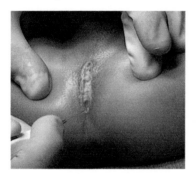 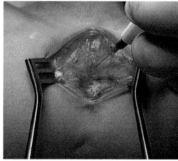

Figure 4.7 Perineal incision in supine position.

PSARP FOR RECTOVESTIBULAR FISTULA

Separating the anterior rectum from the posterior vagina during a rectovestibular fistula dissection can be challenging. A nice maneuver is to first dissect high on the lateral walls of the rectum and only then come across in the area where the anterior rectum and posterior vagina are separate. Passing across a vessel loop provides traction which facilitates the dissection of the distal rectal fistula (Figure 4.8). A new modification avoids any incision of the perineal body.

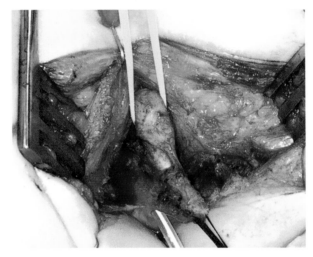

Figure 4.8

RECOMMENDED READING

Badillo AT, Tiusaba L, Jacobs SE, Al-Shamaileh T, Feng C, Russell TL, Bokova E, Sandler AD, Levitt MA. Sparing the Perineal Body - A Modification of the Posterior Sagittal Anorectoplasty (PSARP) for Anorectal Malformations with Rectovestibular Fistulae. *Eur J Pediatr Surg.* [In Press]

FEMALE ANORECTAL MALFORMATION WITH A LOW RECTUM AND NO FISTULA

A female patient with Down syndrome, an ARM, a normal urethra, and a normal introitus was born at 32 weeks' gestation, weighing 1300 grams. There was no visible perineal fistula and no stool at the perineum. The appearance of the perineum and a cross table lateral film is shown in Figure 4.9.

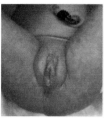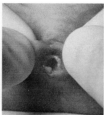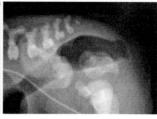

Figure 4.9

What treatment plan would you choose?
   (a)   Primary repair?
   (b)   Colostomy, future distal colostogram, and definitive repair?

Taking into consideration that the child has Down syndrome and a low rectum, a primary anoplasty (see Figure 4.10) would mean less surgery and, hence, is a better treatment choice than a colostomy, a future repair, and a colostomy closure. This is provided, of course, that the baby is well, with no associated comorbidities. A primary surgery is rather challenging in such a small baby, but a colostomy placement and closure are associated with potential additional morbidity. So, both options should be considered. In this case, a primary anoplasty (shown in Figure 4.10) was performed.

> When your cases are never presented during the morbidity and mortality meeting, you are not operating enough.
>
> **– Contributed by:**
> **Martin Lacher**

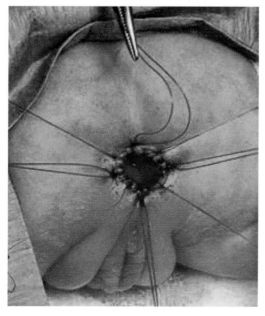

Figure 4.10

RECTOVESTIBULAR FISTULA WITH DISTAL VAGINAL ATRESIA

A full-term newborn has an ARM. The infant was taken to the OR on the first day of life for a PSARP, but, following careful inspection, the perineal exam revealed the findings shown in Figure 4.11.

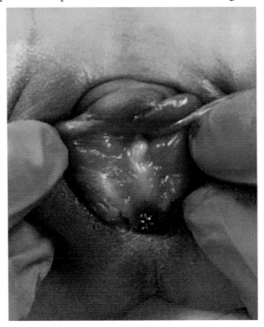

Figure 4.11

It was decided to perform a diagnostic laparoscopy as a first step.

How would you describe the anorectal malformation based on the perineal exam?

The newborn has a rectovestibular fistula, but with an associated distal vaginal atresia. The urethra is normal.

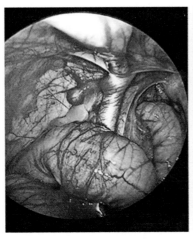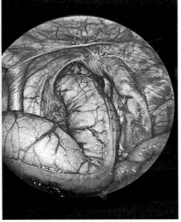

Figure 4.12

What do you see in the laparoscopic images in Figure 4.12?

The findings demonstrated on laparoscopy with inspection of Mullerian structures aid in determining gynecologic options and the surgical approach. In this child, the left Mullerian system is atretic while the right appears normal, allowing for a future vaginal pull-through. Both ovaries are normal (Figure 4.13).

> Without the data the chatta don't matta.
>
> **– Michael Caty**

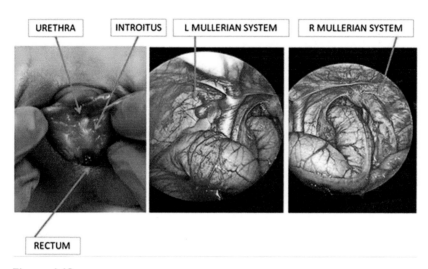

Figure 4.13

Therefore, the surgical plan was to perform a PSARP with vaginal pull-through of the right side and removal of the left atretic system, including the left tube (this reduces the risk of ovarian cancer), with preservation of the ovary. The vaginal pull-through can be done at the same time or delayed until puberty. This case is quite rare because most such cases have no Mullerian structure at all, and the decision needs to be between in such a case, future dilations of the introitus to make a vagina can be done. Laparoscopy is a key step to define the anatomy.

NEWBORN FEMALE WITH AN ANORECTAL MALFORMATION AND NO VISIBLE FISTULA

Kindness begins with the understanding that we all struggle.

– Charles Glassman

This baby girl has an ARM, normal urethra, normal introitus, and no visible fistula. The perineal exam and the distal colostogram are seen in Figure 4.14.

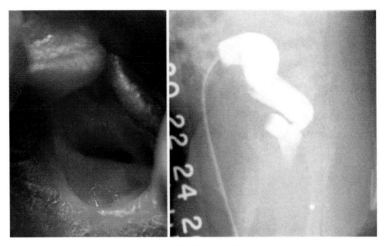

Figure 4.14 (a) Perineal exam, (b) Distal colostogram

What would be your plan for the patient?

Given that there are two perineal openings without a visible rectum, this is an ARM with a recto-vaginal fistula. The height of the rectum as it enters the vagina dictates whether a PSARP or laparoscopic approach would be preferred. A colostomy is needed, and thereafter a distal colostogram will show the rectum. Here the rectum is high on the vaginal dome. Also, a vaginoscopy should be performed to see if there is a vaginal septum, which could be resected at the same time.

CHAPTER 5

ANAL STENOSIS, RECTAL ATRESIA, AND PRESACRAL MASS

MANAGEMENT OF CONGENITAL ANAL STENOSIS

A 7-month-old male with constipation is referred to you by a gastroenterologist who felt the anus was narrow (shown in Figure 5.1). You confirm this on your exam both digitally and using Hegar dilators. There is a firm, circular ridge just inside the anal canal. The contrast study (shown in Figure 5.1) shows significant proximal rectal dilatation.

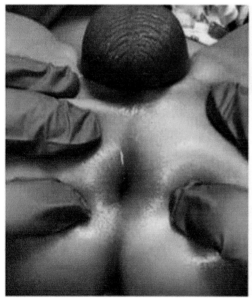 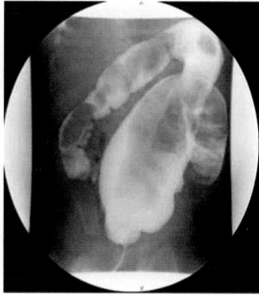

Figure 5.1 Management of anal stenosis.

This is a relatively common referral from a pediatrician to a surgeon, where a digital exam leads to concern about a narrow anal opening. The vast majority of these are normal and need no intervention. Confirmation is necessary, which can be done using sized Hegar dilators. A newborn should be a size 12 Hegar, and 1-year-old a size 15. A digital exam is a must as using Hegar dilators only may miss the feel of the stenotic area that the finger can detect.

Are there any additional radiologic studies needed?
Once true anal stenosis is confirmed, you need to rule out Currarino syndrome in these patients by getting a pelvic MRI to look for a presacral mass (Figure 5.2). The patient will also need a spinal MRI as part of a VACTERL workup and genetic testing.

Would you offer surgery for this patient?
Something needs to be done for this stenosis or it will remain narrow as the child grows and become a worsening obstructive problem.

DOI: 10.1201/9781003150015-6

> You find peace not by rearranging the circumstances of your life, but by realizing who you are at the deepest level.
>
> **– Eckhart Tolle**

Are dilations an option?

Treating anal stenosis with anal dilations is usually not a permanent solution, as the dilations only disrupt the stenosis temporarily, and the stenosis will subsequently re-form.

Would you do a stoma as the first step? Or at the time of the anal surgery?

Stomal diversion should be based on how much anal work is required. If there is a posterior sagittal incision behind the anoplasty, then yes, diversion is needed, likely at the time of the anal repair. However, diversion should take place in advance if the colon is particularly dilated or there are other medical reasons to delay the anoplasty.

If no stoma was required, when would you feed postoperatively?

If only the anus is fixed and there is no incision posteriorly, then feeds can be advanced right away. However, if there is an incision posteriorly, fecal diversion is needed and then feeds can be started right away because there is a stoma.

What surgery should be done?

If the narrowing is long (greater than 3 mm), a repair of the anal stenosis is needed. Repair for a long anal stenosis involves a posterior sagittal incision and mobilization of the posterior rectum to enlarge the anus (Figure 5.4). For a very short area of narrowing (less than or equal to 3 mm), an HM anoplasty will work.

RECOMMENDED READING

Lawal TA, Reck CA, Wood RJ, Lane VA, Gasior A, Diefenbach K, Levitt MA. A modification of the Heineke–Mikulicz concept applied to the treatment of congenital anal stenosis. *J Laparoendosc Adv Surg Tech & Part B Videoscop.* March 2016.

PRESACRAL MASS AND CONSTIPATION

A 5-year-old girl diagnosed at birth with anal stenosis was treated with dilations only. The patient continued to have severe constipation. To treat this, the surgeons caring for her did a sigmoid resection, but the constipation only minimally improved. On evaluation during a second opinion, given the original anorectal diagnosis, an MRI

> Anyone who enjoys inner peace is no more broken by failure than he is inflated by success.
>
> **– Matthieu Ricard**

was done to screen for Currarino syndrome and revealed the presacral mass shown in Figure 5.2. This was not known about or even suspected previously. On digital rectal exam, this mass was palpable and compressed the rectal lumen. The anus has no stenosis anymore; dilations were successful.

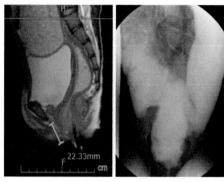

Figure 5.2

How would you manage this patient?
(a) Mass resection alone.
(b) Mass resection plus revision to enlarge the anus.
(c) Mass resection plus colon resection.
(d) Mass resection plus colon resection plus Malone.

There are several learning points within this case:

1. For all anal stenosis (and rectal atresia) cases, an evaluation for a presacral mass is required.
2. All presacral masses need to be assessed by spinal MRI for a dural component. If present, neurosurgery should be involved.
3. If Currarino syndrome is proven, genetic testing of family members is needed.
4. For surgical management, removal of the mass is key and will likely solve much of the constipation.
5. If the anus is narrow, it must be surgically treated with an anal canal sparing technique (Figure 5.4). Dilations alone might succeed, but often the stenosis comes back if the dilations are stopped.
6. With mass removal, the colon should decompress, but an antegrade flush with a Malone might be a helpful adjunct, to help rehabilitate the colon.
7. Whether the colon will recover is a key question. It is better to avoid colonic resection in the primary surgery in the hope that the colon will improve after removing the distal obstruction.
8. A presacral mass, if found, is usually a teratoma. An alpha fetoprotein level should be checked prior to surgery and followed up after resection.

RECOMMENDED READING

Köchling J, et al. The Currarino syndrome-hereditary transmitted syndrome of anorectal, sacral and presacral anomalies. Case report and review of the literature. *Eur J Pediatr Surg.* 1996 April; 6(2): 114–119.

PRESERVING THE ANAL CANAL IN RECTAL ATRESIA AND ANAL STENOSIS

Rectal atresia and anal stenosis are unique ARMs, as the anal canal is present in both and should be preserved. To do this requires understanding two maneuvers, described below:

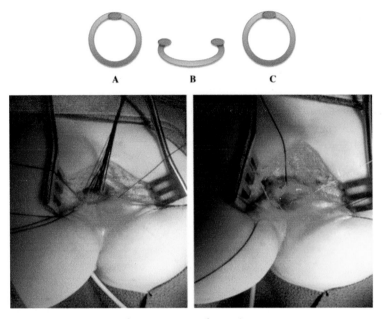

Figure 5.3 Maneuver for treatment of rectal atresia.

In the case of rectal atresia, the anal canal is split along the posterior midline, the distal rectum is mobilized, and then a circle (the lumen of the distal rectum) is sewn to the circle of the now split anal canal. Sutures are placed to recreate the circle (Figure 5.3).

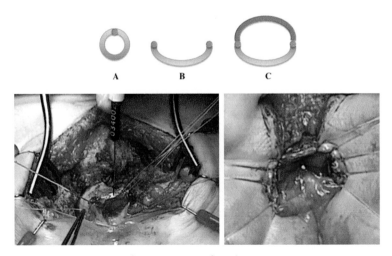

Figure 5.4 Maneuver for treatment of anal stenosis.

In the case of anal stenosis, the anal canal is split along the posterior midline, the distal rectum is mobilized, and then a circle (the lumen of the distal rectum) is sewn to the semicircle of the now split anal canal and to the anal skin posteriorly (Figure 5.4). This is required because the anal canal was too narrow to start. Thus, the final anoplasty has the dentate line on the anterior semicircumference, and the posterior anoplasty is bowel wall sutured to skin.

You deserve to rest. Even if only for a moment. Put down the weight you're carrying. Let go of the need to keep it all together. Take off your warrior mask. For this moment, now … just breathe.

**– Contributed by:
Julie Choueiki, USA**

RECOMMENDED READING

Lane VA, Wood RJ, Reck C, Skerritt C, Levitt MA. Rectal atresia and anal stenosis: The difference in the operative technique for these two distinct congenital anorectal malformations. *Tech Coloproctol.* 2016 Apr; 20(4): 249–254.

PRESACRAL MASS

A patient presents with an opening behind a normal-appearing anus (Figure 5.5).

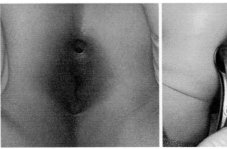

Figure 5.5

What do you think about this case?

This appears to be a rectal duplication, which can be excised via a posterior sagittal incision. Further workup (Figure 5.6) also shows a hemisacrum, a presacral mass (a meningocele), i.e. a case of Currarino triad.

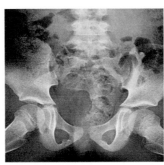

Figure 5.6

How would you approach this repair?

Don't ask if the patient is too sick to have an operation but rather if the patient is too sick to not have an operation.

– Contributed by: Marc Levitt

In this case, a neurosurgeon should be engaged early in the meningocele decision making. In a case of anal stenosis or rectal atresia or, as in this case, what appears to be a rectal duplication, a pelvic and spinal MRI should be obtained. You need to know whether there is any connection of the mass to the dura (or, in this case, if the mass is actually spinal in origin). The most common presacral mass is a teratoma and about 40% of them have a dural connection. You also do not want to inadvertently discover that a tethered cord is exiting the dura during your presacral teratoma resection.

How would your plan change if this was anal stenosis or rectal atresia?

If the anal anomaly were more complicated, such as anal stenosis or rectal atresia, a colostomy would be preferred owing to increased tension on the anoplasty. If there is a presacral mass like a teratoma with no neural connection, this can be resected at the time of the rectal work. But, if the mass is spinal or has any spinal connection/origin, it should be resected separately from any colorectal work to prevent seeding the cerebrospinal fluid, and the operation should be performed in conjunction with neurosurgery.

CHAPTER 6

CLOACA

A CLOACA WITH HYDROCOLPOS

A fetus is suspected prenatally to have a cloaca because of the female gender with a pelvic mass (with a septum) and bilateral hydronephrosis (Figure 6.1).

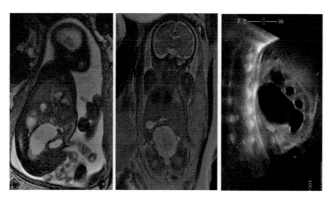

Figure 6.1 Fetal MRI of a cloaca with hydrocolpos.

At birth, the patient had impressive abdominal distension with bilateral hydronephrosis and hydrocolpos.

How would you manage the hydrocolpos?
(a) Intermittent catheterization to drain the vagina.
(b) Vaginostomy using a tube.
(c) Vaginostomy sewn to the abdominal wall.

Intermittent catheterization of the common channel may be therapeutic and should be tried first, as it almost always works, and a surgical decompression (such as a vaginostomy) is not needed. It is important to have the family do the catheterization under ultrasound guidance to be certain they are achieving reliable and reproducible decompression and resolution of the hydronephrosis. A Coudé catheter helps direct the drainage of a right- and a left-sided hydrocolpos. The patient definitely does not need a vesicostomy, as that will not solve the problem, because the hydrocolpos compresses the distal ureters, and a vesicostomy will not relieve the obstruction. If catheterization fails, a formal vaginostomy is necessary. If the hydrocolpos is large, it can be sutured to the abdominal wall like a vesicostomy, or a pigtail tube can be placed. Straight tubes are problematic, because as the hydrocolpos recedes from the anterior abdominal wall over time, the tube will often fall out. If the vagina is surgically drained, the dome of the vagina must be opened and a section of the septum removed, so the two sides can communicate and adequate drainage can be achieved (Figures 6.2 and 6.3).

What is success? To laugh often and much; to win the respect of intelligent people and the affection of children; to earn the appreciation of honest critics and endure the betrayal of false friends; to appreciate the beauty; to find the best in others; to leave the world a bit better, whether by a healthy child, a garden patch or a redeemed social condition; to know even one life has breathed easier because you have lived. This is to have succeeded!

– Ralph Waldo Emerson

DOI: 10.1201/9781003150015-7

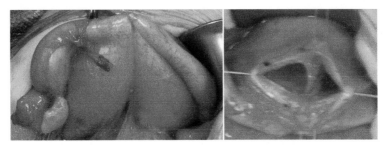

Figure 6.2 Intraoperative picture of vaginal septum in a patient with cloaca and hydrocolpos.

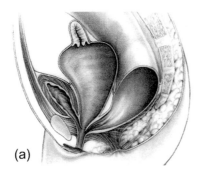
(a)

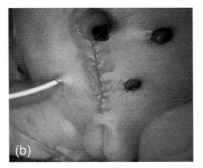
(b)

Figure 6.3 A. Artistic drawing of a cloaca with hydrocolpos. B. In this, a different case, a mid line laparotomy was done with vaginostomy tube and double barrel colostomy.

Case continued: At the time of colostomy creation, it was noticed that the distal colon entered very high on the dome of the vagina, and the rectovaginal fistula was easily visible.

Based on this finding, what type of stoma would you create?

If the end of the bowel enters the dome of the vagina (a very rare circumstance), it is best to do an end stoma rather than a divided colostomy. An end stoma has the advantage of preventing contamination, which usually happens if there is still communication of the distal colon with the urinary tract. Also, this technique will preserve all the arcades for both a future vaginal reconstruction (if one is needed) and for the colonic pull-through. These patients will require a combined abdominal and perineal approach to their operation for the reconstruction anyway. The end of the stoma will become the rectal pull-through in the future and the vaginal replacement if one is needed.

Ten days after end colostomy placement, this patient developed an ileus with no stoma output. The colon became distended, and an ultrasound revealed diffuse ascites.

What might be the etiology of the ascites? What is your plan?

We decided to pass a catheter into the common channel to empty the bladder and repeated the ultrasound. Surprisingly, there was no ascites present anymore. It appeared that the rectovaginal fistula repair had broken down where the distal rectum had been separated from the vaginal dome, and the child was leaking urine from the bladder into the vagina and then into the abdomen. We placed a Foley balloon into the bladder by cystoscopy. Keeping the bladder decompressed allowed the vaginal hole to heal.

CLOACA WITH AN ATYPICAL PELVIC MASS

A baby with a typical cloacal appearance and a large, prenatally diagnosed abdominal mass was admitted to the NICU. Perineal catheterization failed to decompress the mass. It was also unclear on ultrasound what the mass was, although a hydrocolpos was suspected. However, there was, confusingly, no hydronephrosis. The baby was taken to the OR for creation of a colostomy and possible hydrocolpos drainage. In the OR, a massively dilated sigmoid filled with urine and meconium was identified (Figure 6.4). There was no hydrocolpos. Catheterization of the common channel was not difficult. The distal rectum ended at the dome between the two hemivaginas, and there was a bicornuate uterus.

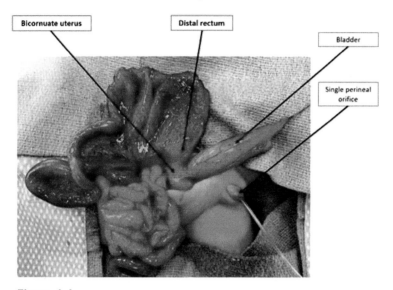

Figure 6.4

What would you do?

The key question here is why there was no hydronephrosis present. If there is a relevant hydrocolpos which may require decompression, there must be associated hydronephrosis.

Interestingly, in this case, the urine went into the sigmoid colon instead of flowing out of the common channel into the vagina(s) and causing a hydrocolpos, which is the more typical scenario. We decompressed the massively dilated sigmoid with a colostomy and irrigated it.

Is any urinary drainage needed in addition to the catheter?

As it was possible to catheterize the common channel, we left a Foley catheter in the bladder and expected the bladder to be able to empty on its own or be catheterized if urine passage was not sufficient.

What type of stoma would you create?

For the colon, we decided that since the distal rectum was preferentially getting the backflow of urine and entered high on the dome of the vagina(s), these structures needed to be separated. So, we closed the rectovaginal fistula and made an end stoma to be the future anoplasty.

Would you do anything about the dilated rectosigmoid?

Because of massive dilation of the sigmoid colon, it was decided to taper it without doing a resection, as this part of the colon might be needed for a vaginal replacement in the future.

CYSTOSCOPY IN A CLOACA TO CATHETERIZE THE BLADDER

It always seems impossible until it is done.

– Nelson Mandela

To gain access to the bladder, cytoscope the common channel and urethra and pass a wire into the bladder. Then, a council tip catheter with a hole at the tip can be passed over that wire. If a council tip catheter is unavailable, a Foley catheter can be used with a little manipulation. First, a large angiocath is placed through the side port of the Foley and out the end, creating a hole. The wire is then passed through the angiocath and the angiocath is removed, leaving the wire in place. The wire is backed out until it goes through the side port, then advanced retrograde through the rest of the catheter. The Foley can then be inserted during cystoscopy (Figure 6.5).

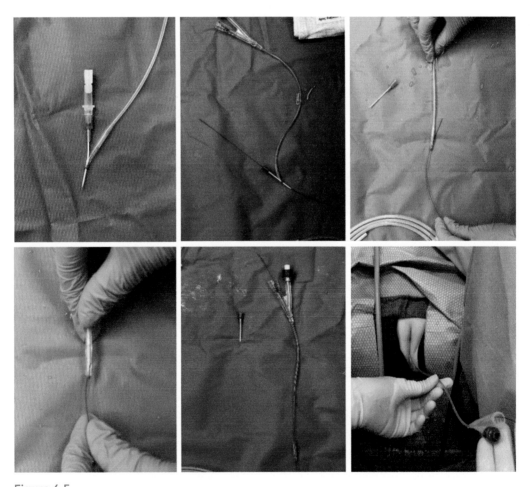

Figure 6.5

CHAPTER 7

POSTOPERATIVE CARE OF A PSARP INCISION

ACTIVITY

After a PSARP, the incision requires delicate care for the best healing outcome. Precautions to consider would be any activity that may be stressful to the perineal area. Consider the patient's age and the activities for their age. An infant should not be carried on the hip of their caregiver, be put in straddling chest/back carriers, or be placed in activity gyms with bounce seats that they straddle. Toys with sharp corners should be removed from the house so there is no accidental sitting on them.

Aim for success, not perfection. Never give up your right to be wrong, because then you will lose the ability to learn new things and move forward with your life.

– David M. Burns

Older children should avoid straddle activities such as bicycle/horseback riding that place pressure on the perineum. To help with these precautions, consider having the diaper-aged patients wear two diapers for 1 month to provide added protection of the perineum (Figure 7.1).

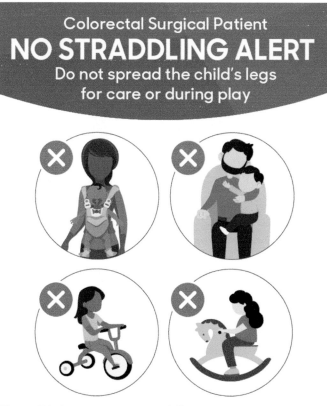

Figure 7.1 Activity precautions following PSARP.

DOI: 10.1201/9781003150015-8

INCISION

For cleaning the incision, avoid tub soaking to prevent the dissolving of the absorbable sutures and separation of the incision. If the patient is old enough to shower, they may do so. Cleaning a young child's incision can include dabbing with moistened gauze or a soft cloth. The incision can also be cleaned by applying water with a peri-bottle, syringe, or handheld bath sprayer. Never rub the incision. If skin breakdown around the incision is present, allow the child's bottom to air dry as much as possible.

SKIN

"But what if I make a mistake?" he asked. She threw back her head and laughed. "A mistake? One mistake? You should be so lucky. You'll make dozens! I made four or five on my first day alone! Of course you'll make mistakes. Just don't make any of them twice. If you do mess things up, don't try to hide it. Don't try to rationalize it. Recognize it and admit it and learn from it. We never stop learning, none of us."

– **John Flanagan**, *Erak's Ransom*

Avoid applying any diaper cream directly to the PSARP incision, but it can be used on the surrounding skin to prevent breakdown. If using antibacterial ointment on the PSARP incision, be sure to educate the parent to use the ointment in moderation and for a short duration. This will help to prevent over-moistening and dissolving of the sutures, which can lead to separation of the PSARP incision. Additionally, parents and the bedside nurses should be cautioned to avoid spreading the buttocks and labia for routine checks. The constant spreading will cause stress on the incision and increase the chance of dehiscence.

FOLEY

If a Foley catheter remains in place for a period of time, be sure to educate the parents on proper Foley care, consistent with your institutional guidelines. Care instructions should include Foley cleaning as well as maintenance of catheter patency. Using a double diaper with the Foley draining into the outer diaper keeps the patient dry and minimizes the risk of inadvertent tugging of the catheter.

PAIN MANAGEMENT

Owing to the midline nature of the PSARP incision, this procedure typically is very tolerable pain-wise with only mild discomfort. However, pain and comfort considerations need to start at the time of the procedure. Patients typically only need a few days of IV pain medication and can quickly transition to oral pain coverage. At discharge, typically only very mild pain control is needed. If the PSARP was accompanied by an abdominal approach, more coverage may be required.

CHAPTER 8

RARE CASES

AN ANORECTAL MALFORMATION WITH A RARE ASSOCIATED UROLOGIC ANOMALY

A newborn with an ARM is shown in Figure 8.1.

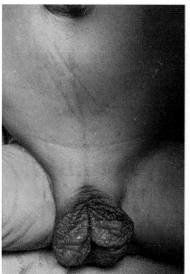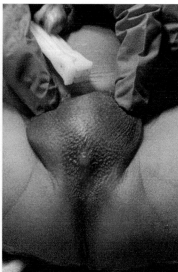

Figure 8.1 ARM with a rare associated urologic anomaly.

What urologic anomaly is this?

This is a very rare case of aphallia with an imperforate anus.

What newborn intervention would you do?

The patient should undergo the usual VACTERL screening and chromatin Y testing. In the newborn period, the baby needs a colostomy and a urinary diversion (suprapubic tube or a vesicostomy).

> Do things for people not because of who they are or what they do in return, but because of who you are.
>
> **– Harold S. Kushner**

What are his future reconstructive needs?

In the next few months, after performing a colostogram to determine the distal rectal anatomy, the patient will need a PSARP followed by a colostomy closure. A neophallus creation will be in his distant future, and the urologic reconstruction for this could include: neophalloplasty, urethroplasty, prosthetic implant, and Mitrofanoff.

RECOMMENDED READING

Gabler T, Charlton R, Loveland J, Mapunda E. Aphallia: A review to standardize management. *Pediatr Surg Int.* 2018 Aug; 34(8): 813–821.

DOI: 10.1201/9781003150015-9

COLONIC TRIPLICATION IN A PATIENT WITH AN ANORECTAL MALFORMATION

A male infant born with an ARM is taken to the operating room for a colostomy and mucus fistula creation. He is found to have three proximal colonic lumens and two distal lumens when the sigmoid is transected. The patient is now 8 months old. The three proximal lumens and a prolapsed mucus fistula are present on the abdomen (Figure 8.2).

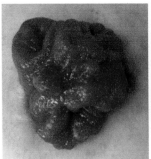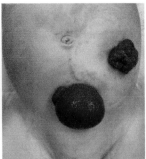

Figure 8.2 Three proximal lumens and a prolapsed mucus fistula with 2 lumens.

Don't lose yourself in the chaos. If life starts moving too fast, put up a fight. Fight back with your bare feet on the earth, fight back by looking up at the stars … or watching a sunset. Fight back by creating space to be still and breathe.

– **Brooke Hampton**

High resolution contrast and 3D imaging were obtained (Figure 8.3). The mucus fistula had one blind-ending lumen while the other fistulized to the posterior bladder. The colostomy had three lumens which transitioned to two lumens just prior to the transverse colon. The duplication continued through to the cecum.

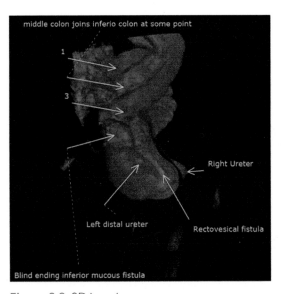

Figure 8.3 3D imaging.

An ileal duplication and fused appendiceal duplication were also identified intraoperatively (Figure 8.4).

Intraluminal stapling was performed to create a single lumen in the ascending and descending colons to aid in future bowel management and to create a unified channel for antegrade flow if the patient needed a Malone. A PSARP was performed to separate the rectovesical fistula and unify the two distal rectums, the colostomy was closed, the ileal duplication was resected, and a diverting ileostomy was created (Figure 8.5).

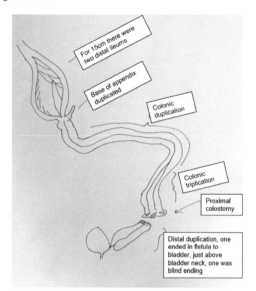

Figure 8.4 Diagram of operative findings.

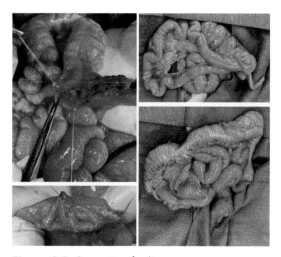

Figure 8.5 Operative findings.

Learning Points:

1. Initial diversion was the correct move in the manner it was performed.
2. At reconstruction, creating a single distal rectum with no communication with the urinary tract is vital.
3. Planning for the future, given the possibility that this patient may require antegrade flushes, a single lumen that can be flushed using a Malone is key. Therefore, we made a common channel at the start and at the end of the colon.

RECOMMENDED READING

McKenna E, Ho C, Badillo A, Villalona G, Levitt M. A rare case of colonic triplication with associated imperforate anus in a newborn male. *European J Pediatr Surg Rep.* [In Press]

CLOACAL EXSTROPHY WITH A GIANT OMPHALOCELE

A 32-week premature baby with cloacal exstrophy who weighs 1.7 kg at birth is in the NICU. She has a giant omphalocele containing her liver shown in Figure 8.6.

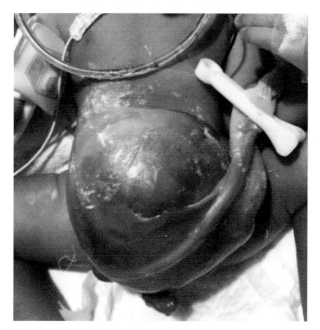

Figure 8.6

How would you manage this patient?

The child has a low birth weight and is small compared to the size of the omphalocele. We suggest applying Silvadene paint to the omphalocele and hydrogel dressings to the exstrophy portion and waiting for the patient to grow prior to the surgical repair. The stool and urine can just leak onto the perineum and be managed without diversion.

Before the age of 3 months, she was successfully fed through a nasogastric tube, stool was drained from the cecal plate, and urine was emptied from the bladder halves.

When do you decide to perform a surgical intervention? What operation would you do?

The omphalocele sac completely epithelialized, and the child has grown to 3.7 kg. Owing to the large size of the omphalocele, the abdominal wall could not be closed. The cecal plate and distal ileum remain between the bladder halves.

> Between stimulus and response there is a space. In that space is our power to choose our response. In our response lies our growth and our freedom.
>
> – Viktor Frankl

Leaving the cecal plate and distal ileum untouched does not usually cause acidosis and it also auto-augments the bladder. This strategy is useful for the future reconstruction, as it allows for formation of a larger bladder during the bladderneck and abdominal wall closure that is planned. The traditional approach of separation and tubularization of the cecal plate can thus be avoided. To set up for a future colonic pull-through, an anastomosis between the distal ileum and the hindgut is easier to perform than a cecal tubularization. The distal hindgut can be made into an end stoma.

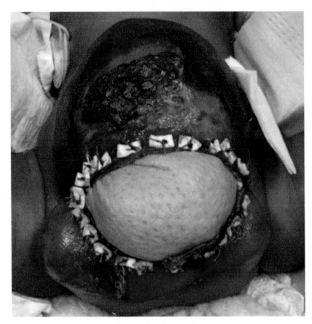

Figure 8.7 Abdominal wall at the conclusion of the operation.

The abdominal wound healed after the operation (Figure 8.7). At the age of 16 months, the omphalocele and bladder exstrophy closure could be done. In the future, if the patient is able to make a solid stool, a colonic pull-through can be considered.

> It is not the strongest of the species that survives, nor the most intelligent. It is the one that is most adaptable.
>
> **– Charles Darwin**

RECOMMENDED READING

Smith CA, Avansino JR, Merguerian P, Lane V, Levitt MA. A novel surgical approach for the management of cloacal exstrophy with a giant omphalocele. *European J Pediatr Surg Rep.* 2021 Jan; 9(1): e41–e45.

CHAPTER 9

ANORECTAL MALFORMATION MYTHS

MYTH: COMMON CHANNEL LENGTH DETERMINES CLOACAL RECONSTRUCTION APPROACH

Formerly it was the length of the common channel in a patient with cloaca that determined the type of cloacal reconstruction procedure, total urogenital mobilization (TUM) or urogenital (UG) separation, to be used for the patient's repair (Figure 9.1). However, it is now clear that the urethral length is also a key factor.

A detailed understanding of the anatomy of a cloacal malformation is critical to the successful repair of these challenging surgical patients. There are multiple components aside from the common channel length to consider, and having an organized approach following anatomic assessment is vital.

> As a single footstep will not make a path on the earth, so a single thought will not make a pathway in the mind. To make a deep physical path, we walk again and again. To make a deep mental path, we must think over and over the kind of thoughts we wish to dominate our lives.
>
> **– Henry David Thoreau**

After the endoscopy, cloacagram, and review of the imaging and the intra-operative findings from the colostomy creation, the surgical team should know the following:

1. The length of the common channel.
2. The length of the urethra.
3. The anatomy of the vagina(s) and sometimes the anatomy of the upper genital tract.
4. The location of the rectal fistula.
5. The location of the true rectum and its position in relation to the PC line.

This information will help predict, plan, and execute a safe and optimal surgical strategy. The reconstruction involves either a TUM or UG separation and is performed according to measurements determined by the factors above.

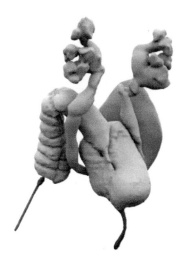

Figure 9.1 Assessing a cloaca for the reconstructive plan.

DOI: 10.1201/9781003150015-10

Sometimes it feels like we are rearranging the deck chairs on the *Titanic*.

– Contributed by: Marc Levitt

The cloacal reconstruction algorithm (see Figure 9.2) considers the role of both the common channel and the urethral lengths in determining surgical planning. A short urethra, less than 1.5 cm, should not be mobilized. This avoids pulling the bladderneck down, below the urogenital diaphragm, which will lead to urinary incontinence.

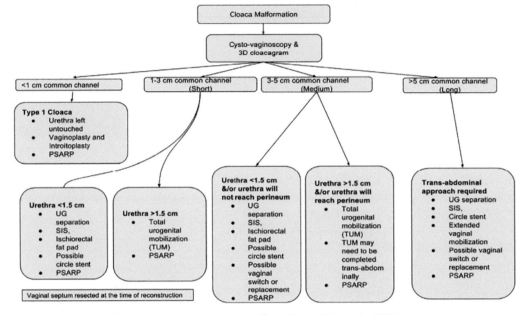

Figure 9.2 Algorithm for cloaca management (from Wood RJ et al., 2017).

RECOMMENDED READING

Halleran DR, Smith CA, Fuller MK, Durhm MM, Dickie B, Avansino JR, Tirrell TF, Vandewalle R, Reeder R, Drake KR, Bates DG, Rollins MD, Levitt MA, Wood RJ, Pediatric Colorectal and Pelvic Learning Consortium. Measure twice and cut once: Comparing endoscopy and 3D cloacagram for the common channel and urethral measurements in patients with cloacal malformations. *J Pediatr Surg.* 2020 Feb; 55(2): 257–260.

Halleran DR, Thompson B, Fuchs M, Vilanova-Sanchez A, Rentea RM, Bates DG, McCracken K, Hewitt G, Ching C, DaJusta D, Levitt MA, Wood RJ. Urethral length in female infants and its relevance in the repair of cloaca. *J Pediatr Surg.* 2019 Feb; 54(2): 303–306.

Reck-Burneo CA, Lane V, Bates DG, Hogan M, Thompson B, Gasior A, Weaver L, Dingemans AJM, Maloof T, Hoover E, Gagnon R, Wood R, Levit M. The use of rotational fluoroscopy and 3-D reconstruction in the diagnosis and surgical planning for complex cloacal malformations. *J Pediatr Surg.* 2019 Aug; 54(8): 1590–1594.

Skerritt C, Wood RJ, Jayanthi VR, Levitt MA, Ching CB, DaJusta DG, Fuchs ME. Does a standardized operative approach in cloacal reconstruction allow for preservation of a patent urethra? *J Pediatr Surg.* 2021 Jan 14; S0022-3468(21): 00031-2.

Wood RJ, Reck-Burneo CA, Dajusta D, Ching C, Jayanthi R, Bates DG, Fuchs ME, McCracken K, Hewitt G, Levitt MA. Cloaca reconstruction: A new algorithm that considers the role of urethral length in determining surgical planning. *J Pediatr Surg.* 2017 Oct 12; S0022-3468(17): 30644-9.

Wood, Richard J., et al. Organizing the care of a patient with a cloacal malformation: Key steps and decision making for pre-, intra-, and post-operative repair. *Semin Pediatr Surg.* 2020 Dec; 9(6).

MYTH: CLOACAL EXSTROPHY MEANS A PERMANENT STOMA

Previously, nearly normal pelvic and sacral anatomy and the presence of normal sphincter mechanisms were thought to be requirements to perform a pull-through operation for children born with cloacal exstrophy (Figure 9.3). However, the indications for a pull-through have expanded and now include successful bowel management through the stoma, which depends on the patient's ability to form solid stool.

Candidates for colonic pull-through include those who can form solid stool (i.e. those with enough colon), have a reasonable degree of pelvic neuromuscular development, and comply with a bowel management program (BMP). The ability to form solid stool is assessed via bowel management involving a constipating diet, antidiarrheals, bulking agents, and a daily enema through the stoma.

Patients who undergo successful bowel management through the stoma are offered a pull-through, and many can remain clean. The key factors are the capacity to form solid stool and the success of a once daily passage of stool in response to an antegrade flush. Otherwise, the patient is best served by a stoma. To maximize pull-through poten-

> Most people do not listen with the intent to understand. Most people listen with the intent to reply.
>
> **– Stephen R. Covey**

tial, it is crucial to use all available hindgut for the initial colostomy and avoid using the colon for urologic or genital reconstruction with the exception of the cecum. Most patients have a poor prognosis for bowel control but are able to remain clean with bowel management via antegrade flushes.

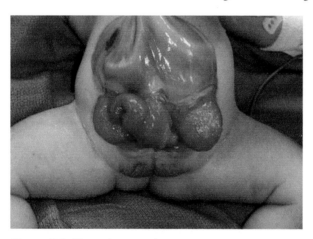

Figure 9.3 Cloacal exstrophy.

RECOMMENDED READING

Levitt MA, Mak GZ, Falcone RA Jr, Peña A. Cloacal exstrophy – pull-through or permanent stoma? A review of 53 patients. *J Pediatr Surg*. 2008 Jan; 43(1): 164–168; discussion 168–170.

Sawaya D, Goldstein S, Seetharamaiah R, Suson K, Nabaweesi R, Colombani P, Gearhart J. Gastrointestinal ramifications of the cloacal exstrophy complex: A 44-year experience. *J Pediatr Surg*. 2010 Jan; 45(1): 171–175; discussion 175–176.

PART II
HIRSCHSPRUNG DISEASE

CHAPTER 10

DIAGNOSIS

SUCTION RECTAL BIOPSY

The suction rectal biopsy gun invented by Helen Noblett from Melbourne, Australia in 1969 is an ingenious device that allows one to obtain a rectal biopsy in infants to diagnose Hirschsprung disease (HD) (Figure 10.1).

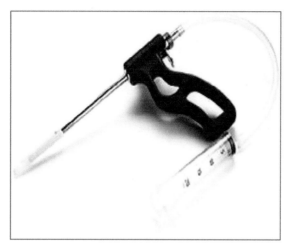

Figure 10.1 Rectal biopsy device.

The device is placed inside the anal verge, and two to three specimens are obtained posteriorly and laterally (Figure 10.2). It is vital to not take the biopsy too high (greater than 3 cm), as you could miss the aganglionosis, or too low, because the anal canal is aganglionic in all patients. Bleeding after the procedure is rare, but if it happens, a digital exam with the fifth digit pressing down on the sacrum stops the bleeding. Additionally, insertion of a tampon/plug created with Surgicel™ (oxidized regenerated cellulose) may be used to control capillary, venous, and small arterial bleeding.

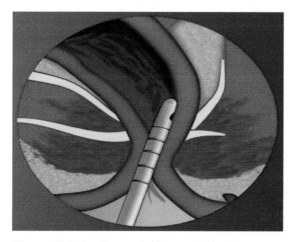

Figure 10.2 Suction rectal biopsy technique.

DOI: 10.1201/9781003150015-12

OPEN FULL-THICKNESS RECTAL BIOPSY

For surgeons, hope is not a strategy.

– Fred Ryckman

An open, full-thickness rectal biopsy is needed for older patients, patients with a previous pull-through, or patients with a previously insufficient suction rectal biopsy. During the exam, the surgeon can identify the dentate line and select where to perform the biopsy. This is especially helpful for redo cases where one must identify the previous anastomosis and perform the biopsy proximal to it.

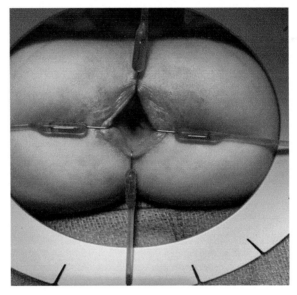

Figure 10.3 Exposure of the anal canal to obtain an open biopsy.

Place the lone star ring and pins to gain good exposure of the dentate line and anal canal (Figure 10.3).

There comes a time in every operation where you have to cut.

– Barry Shandling, Contributed by: Jack Langer

Next, introduce a 4 × 4 sponge through the anal canal to avoid the passage of stool during the procedure. This sponge acts as a "colorectal cork". Tag the cork with a suture and a clamp so you remember to remove it at the procedure's conclusion (Figure 10.4).

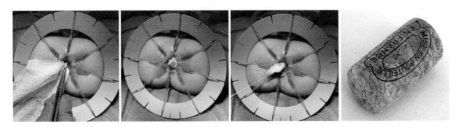

Figure 10.4 The colorectal cork (a sponge) prevents stool from passing during the biopsy procedure.

Place two stay sutures, one proximal to the intended biopsy site, with the needle left attached, and one distal to the planned biopsy site. The proximal suture will be used to close the defect once the biopsy is taken. The distal suture pulls down to show a ridge of colonic mucosa for the biopsy site. To take the biopsy, use tenotomy scissors as they are sharp and help to take an adequate biopsy, including mucosa and submucosa (Figure 10.5). Then, close the defect with a running suture using the initial proximal stitch. Check for hemostasis before taking out the lone star pins and removing the gauze.

> You will spend a lot of time figuring out what to do and spend more time figuring out what not to do.
>
> **– Contributed by:**
> **Mohamed Abdelmalak**

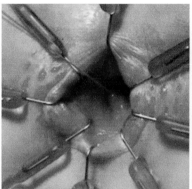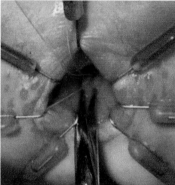

Figure 10.5 Open biopsy technique.

NO GANGLION CELLS AND NO HYPERTROPHIC NERVES: IS THIS HIRSCHSPRUNG DISEASE?

The best operation is the operation you do best.

– Fred Ryckman

For a definitive diagnosis of HD, there must be a histologic absence of ganglion cells and the presence of hypertrophic nerves (greater than 40 μm) in 100 levels of the biopsy.

What does it mean when the pathologist reports no ganglion cells and no presence of hypertrophic nerves?

When the pathologist reports no ganglionic cells and no hypertrophic nerves, it means that the biopsy was probably taken too low. It must be remembered that there is a physiologic aganglionic segment in the anal canal. This was first reported in the Journal of Pediatric Surgery in 1968. One of the original illustrations in the paper is shown in Figure 10.6.

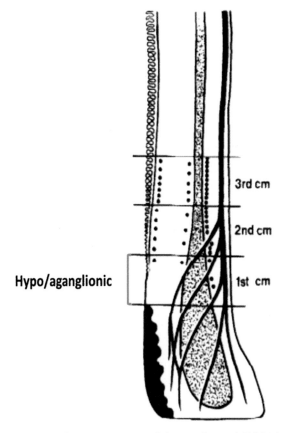

Figure 10.6 Physiologic a aganglionic segment of the anal canal (Aldridge RT & Campbell PE, 1968).

The dots represent the distribution of ganglion cells in the anal canal of healthy people. As you see in the first centimeter proximal to the dentate line, there is a lack of ganglion cells. Because of that we should not be tricked into diagnosing a patient with HD by only noting the absence of ganglion cells.

The distribution of ganglion cells in the colonic wall flows like paint dripping down the sides of a can. So, one could biopsy between the drips and find no ganglion cells (Figure 10.7). This is particularly relevant when biopsying a patient with a previous pull-through.

> More harm came because you did not look than from not knowing what was in the book.
>
> **– Michael Klein**

To summarize the interpretation of a full-thickness rectal biopsy on pathologic reports in a variety of scenarios:

1. No ganglion cells only – not enough information.
2. No ganglion cells plus hypertrophic nerves – consistent with HD.
3. No ganglion cells and normal-sized nerves – likely a sampling error.
4. No ganglion cells plus squamous epithelium – biopsy was taken too low.
5. Ganglion cells with hypertrophic nerves – consistent with constipation (hypertrophy of nerves is secondary to rectal stretch).
6. Ganglion cells with eosinophils – this could be explained by a milk protein allergy.

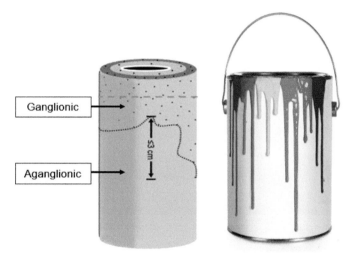

Figure 10.7

RECOMMENDED READING

Aldridge RT, Campbell PE. Ganglion cell distribution in the normal rectum and anal canal. A basis for the diagnosis of Hirschsprung's disease by anorectal biopsy. *J Pediatr Surg*. 1968 Aug; 3(4): 475–490.

EXTRACORPOREAL FULL-THICKNESS BIOPSY DURING LAPAROSCOPIC-ASSISTED PULL-THROUGH

When performing leveling biopsies for a laparoscopic pull-through, extracorporeal biopsies are easier, faster, and less likely to cause intra-abdominal contamination. Once you have moved the camera to the right upper quadrant, select the piece of bowel that is likely to be proximal to the aganglionic segment based on the contrast enema. Insert the grasper through the umbilicus. Then pull that piece of bowel out through the umbilical port and take a full-thickness biopsy (Figure 10.8).

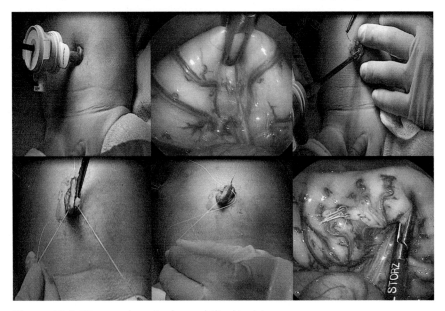

Figure 10.8 Biopsy taken via the umbilical incision.

This biopsy should be a cube with the square of mucosa the same size as the square of the seromuscular layer. This is affectionately called a "Tiusaba biopsy". The biopsy size and shape help the pathologist orient the specimen and ensure adequate submucosa for analysis. Close the defect and send the specimen for frozen section analysis. Taking a seromuscular biopsy only, which is a common technique during a laparoscopic pull-through, risks missing that you are in a transition zone because the seromuscular layer could have ganglion cells, but the submucosal layer could have hypertrophic nerves (Figure 10.9).

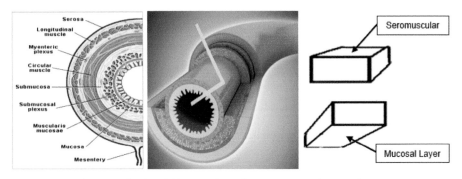

Figure 10.9 The sample should be a cube of tissue, not a diamond.

HEGAR DILATOR TRICK FOR STOMA CREATION AND TRANSUMBILICAL BIOPSY

In countries with limited resources, ileostomies carry a higher morbidity because of the inability to recognize and access treatment for high output due to infectious diarrheal illnesses and Hirschsprung-associated enterocolitis (HAEC). For this reason, if a primary pull-through is not being done, colostomies are preferable in the setting of HD. Stomas for HD need not necessitate a large midline laparotomy. A circular incision can be made in the left lower quadrant where the colon can be delivered and decompressed with an IV cannula to facilitate visualization through the smaller incision (Figure 10.10).

> Specializing helps you learn more and more about less and less until you know everything about nothing.
>
> **– Contributed by: Tarryn Gabler**

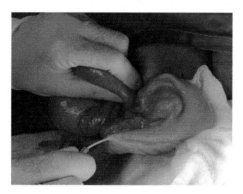

Figure 10.10

Using a Hegar dilator placed through the anus will help identify the proximal and distal parts of the sigmoid colon (Figure 10.11).

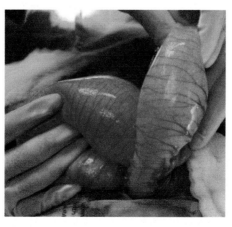

Figure 10.11

In the absence of laparoscopy, this maneuver allows for identification of the sigmoid colon and can also be used to direct the sigmoid up through a small umbilical incision, allowing for full-thickness biopsies to be performed. Biopsy of the sigmoid and transverse colon for colonic mapping of the extent of HD prior to the pull-through can be accomplished through a small umbilical incision.

FROZEN SECTION BIOPSY IN THE MANAGEMENT OF HIRSCHSPRUNG DISEASE

Nothing in life is to be feared, it is only to be understood. Now is the time to understand more, so that we may fear less.

– Marie Curie, Contributed by: Teresa Russell

Though frozen section cannot be used to diagnose HD, it can be used to rule out HD. In other words, you can "rule out" but not "rule in" HD by frozen section. A definitive diagnosis of HD requires 100 sections of tissue, stained with hematoxylin & Eosin (H & E), acetylcholinesterase, or calretinin to identify the necessary features on histology, i.e. the absence of ganglion cells and the presence of hypertrophic nerves (greater than 40 μm). The frozen section only allows time for microscopic evaluation of a limited number of sections to look for ganglion cells. As soon as the pathologist identifies one ganglion cell, HD can be excluded (Figure 10.12).

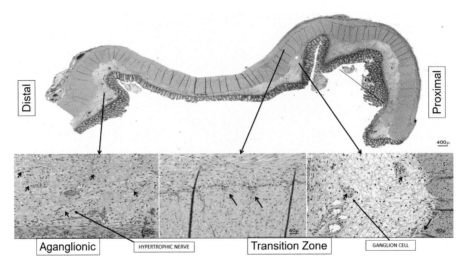

Figure 10.12 Segment of bowel showing aganglionic, transition zone, and normal bowel histology.

CHAPTER 11

THE PULL-THROUGH

A NEWBORN WITH HIRSCHSPRUNG DISEASE UNDERGOES SURGERY

A newborn presents with abdominal distension, and HD is proven by rectal biopsy. Irrigations have been somewhat successful, but the baby remains distended. His contrast study is shown in Figure 11.1.

> When someone who is blind sees something, it is probably there.
>
> **– Alberto Peña**

Is the patient ready for definitive surgery?
Which option below should be the next step?

(a) You can continue the irrigations and plan for elective outpatient surgery.

(b) From the contrast enema, the patient appears to have a transition zone at the splenic flexure. A pull-through with a frozen section can be performed.

(c) The patient needs colonic biopsies and a leveling colostomy or ileostomy.

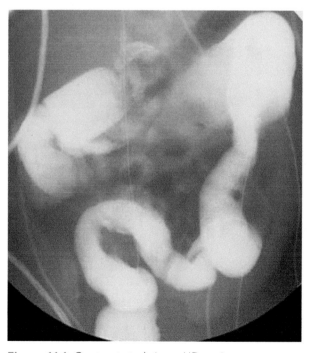

Figure 11.1 Contrast study in an HD patient.

The transition zone is likely at the splenic flexure. Remember that the contrast study is only a guide and can incorrectly estimate the location of the transition zone in 10% of cases. Irrigations have only been somewhat successful, which is a clue that there is limited control of this situation. The transition zone is likely more proximal than the sigmoid, and the irrigation tube does not reach the dilated bowel.

DOI: 10.1201/9781003150015-13

> There's a snake under every rock.
>
> **– Michael Caty**

The patient needs colonic mapping with a leveling colostomy in the dilated portion of the bowel (ideally confirmed by frozen section if available) or a diverting ileostomy to decompress the colon. If you map the colon with biopsies, make sure to mark each biopsy site with a permanent suture so these locations can be found in the future. Frozen section analysis that is proximal to the splenic flexure should not be depended upon. The permanent sections are more accurate. The presence of ganglion cells anywhere in the colon is reliable if you have good frozen section capacity, but hypertrophic nerves are not really present proximal to the left colon (no more impact from the sacral plexus), so confirming that you are in a zone of good bowel is not obvious until you have results of the permanent specimens. If no ganglion cells are identified at the left colon, a primary pull-through should not be performed. Permanent specimen analysis is needed to confirm the level.

Also, from a technical point of view, if the transition zone is proximal to the splenic flexure, you need to be prepared to do a colonic derotation. A colonic derotation brings the pull-through down the right side with the entire small bowel placed on the left side.

RECOMMENDED READING

Proctor ML, Traubici J, Langer JC, et al. Correlation between radiographic transition zone and level of aganglionosis in Hirschsprung's disease: Implications for surgical approach. *J Pediatr Surg.* 2003 May; 38(5): 775–778.v

WHERE WOULD YOU START THE TRANSANAL DISSECTION IN A HIRSCHSPRUNG CASE?

The dissection is best started 0.5 cm proximal to the top of the crypts, to ensure the preservation of the dentate line. Its preservation and avoidance of overspreading of the sphincters are the keys to maintaining the patient's potential for bowel control (Figure 11.2).

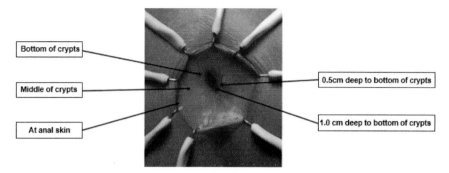

Figure 11.2 View of the transanal approach with relevant sections labeled.

The pins are placed to show the dentate line and then advanced to hide and protect the dentate line. The line of dissection (the purple line of Lee) preserves the area 0.5 cm proximal to the anal canal, which is vital for the continence mechanism. After the purple line is cut, the pins are advanced into that cut line to assist with the dissection.

The transanal dissection is shown in Figure 11.3. In the left image, the dentate line is visible; in the middle image, the dentate line is now hidden; and in the right, the purple line shows the planned dissection. Figure 11.4 shows another view of the purple line of Lee along with Dr. Lee, for whom it is named, alongside Dr. Levitt.

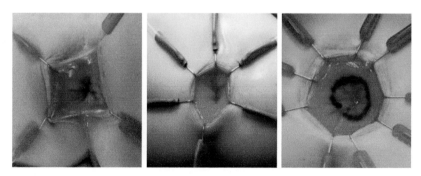

Figure 11.3 Transanal dissection.

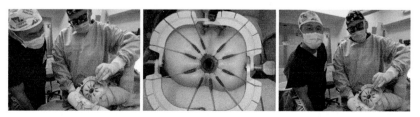

Figure 11.4 View of the "purple line of Lee," shown here with Dr. Levitt and Dr. Timothy Lee himself, after whom the line is named.

SHOWING THE VESSELS TO HELP MOBILIZE THE DISTAL BOWEL VIA A TRANSANAL-ONLY APPROACH

To gain length on the distal pull-through during a primary or redo case via a transanal approach, a nice trick is to grasp the bowel with your fingers through a piece of gauze (Figure 11.5). This allows the surgeon to produce some tension on the bowel's posterior wall and to see the vessels that are holding the bowel in the pelvis. Gently twirl the pull-through in your fingers to show the tension lines, then place a Mixter clamp (shown in Figure 11.6) under the vessels and cauterize them. Before you burn the vessels, relax the bowel so the vessels are not under tension when they are cauterized.

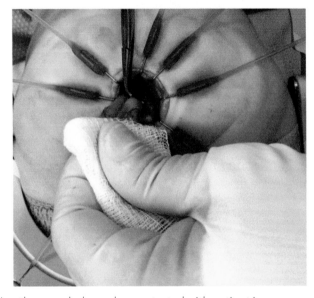

Figure 11.5 Showing the vessels, here demonstrated with patient in prone position.

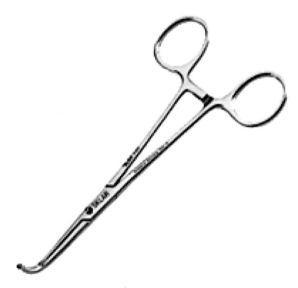

Figure 11.6 Mixter clamp.

WILL THE PULL-THROUGH REACH?

To determine whether a pull-through will reach the perineum, a good landmark is the point 4 cm below the superior edge of the pubic bone. Place a mark at the upper edge of the pubic bone and measure the point 4 cm caudal to this. If the distal rectum reaches to this point, it will reach the anus when the pull-through is passed through the pelvis (Figure 11.7).

> Variability is the law of life ... no two individuals react alike or behave alike under the abnormal conditions which we know as disease.
>
> **– Sir William Osler**

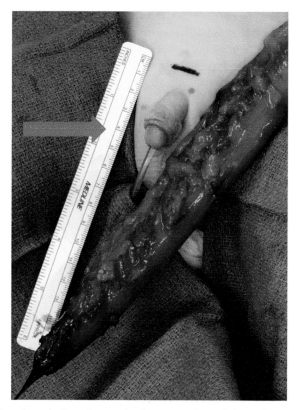

Figure 11.7 Measuring 4 cm below the marked upper edge of the public bone to determine if a patient's pull-through will reach the perineum.

GAINING LENGTH: UNDERSTANDING THE COLONIC ARCADE

In theory, theory and practice are the same. In practice they are not.

– Albert Einstein

To gain length on the colonic mesentery for a pull-through to reach the perineum without tension, it is important to understand which blood vessels can be ligated while preserving the blood supply to the colon.

Imagine the blood vessels are a row of martini glasses. The stems of the glasses act as tether points and serve as a redundant blood supply. The stem of the glass can be ligated, keeping the V of the glass intact. Now imagine the martini glass as a set of strings. When the tethering "stem" is released, the V configuration stretches and flattens to provide additional length. The ligation of the vessel should be done with sutures rather than with cautery to prevent thermal spread. The V represents the intact marginal blood supply through which the vascular supply is maintained (Figure 11.8).

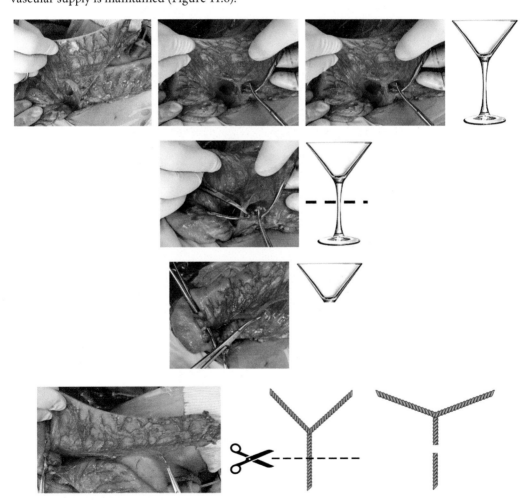

Figure 11.8 Schematic of colonic arcade.

This maneuver is helpful for a colonic pull-through, as well as when one needs to move a segment of the colon for a vaginal or esophageal replacement.

GETTING THE HEPATIC FLEXURE TO REACH WITHOUT CAUSING DUODENAL OBSTRUCTION

For a transition zone at the mid-transverse or hepatic flexure, the colon must be derotated and brought down the right pelvis, with the small bowel placed on the left side of the abdomen. If the pull-through is brought down the left pelvis, the middle colic or the ileocolic artery will kink the third portion of the duodenum and cause obstruction, so this must be avoided. To set up the right colon for this pull-through, the middle and right colic vessels are ligated, and the pull-through is then left to depend on the ileocolic artery and its marginal branch that parallels the right colon. The colon is derotated with the cecum oriented toward the liver and the distal right colon toward the pelvis, and it is brought down the right side of the abdomen (Figures 11.9–11.11).

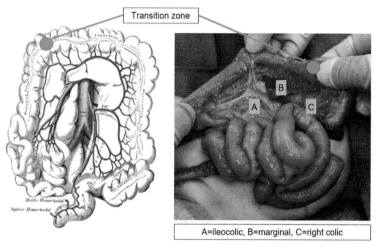

A=ileocolic, B=marginal, C=right colic

Figure 11.9 Defining the arcade for a hepatic flexure transition zone.

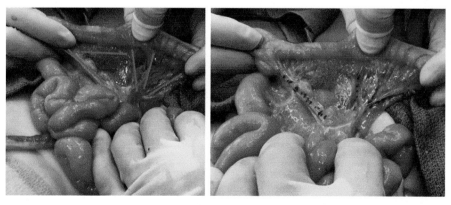

Figure 11.10 Key vessels marked, middle and right colic vessels can be ligated.

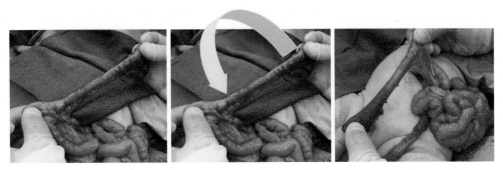

Figure 11.11 Derotation of the colon, the cecum moves to the right upper quadrant and the right colon comes down the right pelvis.

If there is no marginal branch from the ileocolic, the right colic will need to be saved, as seen in Figure 11.12.

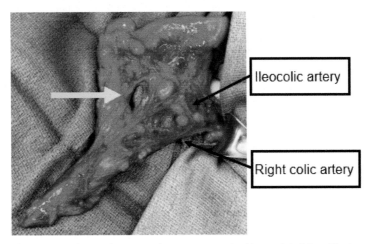

Figure 11.12 Yellow arrow shows the area where no marginal branch is identified, so the right colic must be preserved.

AVOIDING A TWIST OF THE PULL-THROUGH

To avoid a twist in the pull-through, place sutures at the 6 or 12 o'clock positions of the bowel along its longitudinal extent as you progress in the dissection. This maneuver helps to avoid twisting of the pull-through. When the anastomosis is set up, pass a large 24 Fr Foley up into the

> Better to make the important measurable than the measurable important.
>
> **– Contributed by: Jonathan Sutcliffe**

pelvis to again check for a twist. If laparoscopy or laparotomy was used, take a final look at the pull-through to ensure that it is straight and tension free (Figure 11.13).

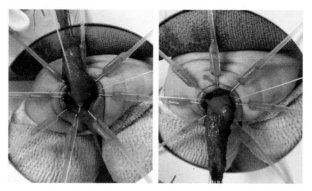

Figure 11.13 Avoiding a twist of the pull-through with a marking suture at 6 or 12 o'clock.

COLO-COLONIC ANASTOMOSIS WITH SIZE DISCREPANCY

It is typical to find a size discrepancy when performing a Hirschsprung pull-through anastomosis. To solve this problem, when sewing a larger circle to a smaller one to create an anastomosis, place sutures at the 3, 6, 9, and 12 o'clock positions, tie down, and tag to mosquito clamps. Then grasp two adjacent mosquitoes, hold them apart, and place a suture to divide the segment of the anastomosis between them. Keep dividing and dividing where you place the stitches, and you will remove any redundancy. This technique can also be used for small bowel to small bowel anastomosis (Figure 11.14).

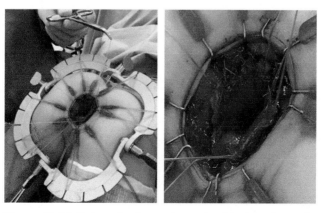

Figure 11.14 Colo-colonic anastomosis with size mismatch.

CHAPTER 12

TOTAL COLONIC HIRSCHSPRUNG DISEASE

TOTAL COLONIC HIRSCHSPRUNG DISEASE

For patients with total colonic HD (TCHD) (Figure 12.1), how do you plan their surgery?

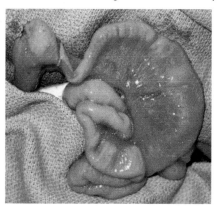

Figure 12.1 Total colonic aganglionosis with transition zone in the ileum.

What are the criteria that the child must meet to schedule the pull-through?
Is there a specific age at which you would perform the pull-through?
What type of pull-through would you perform?

> Do you know what is the most difficult operation? It is the one that you didn't prepare for.
>
> – Jan H. Louw

Answers:

(a) Thickened stool and good growth, with no need for hyperalimentation or supplemental enteral formula. Check urine sodium and keep it above 20 mmol/L. If low, this could explain a stagnation in the patient's growth; they are total body sodium depleted. They need oral sodium to absorb glucose more effectively.

(b) The patient is usually ready sometime between 6 and 18 months. There is no real difference in terms of skin excoriation between patients who are potty trained or not potty trained. Patients over age 4 may hold their sphincters very tightly which can lead to proctalgia (severe anal sphincter spasm), something a baby would not be able to do.

(c) A straight ileoanal pull-through or an ileo-Duhamel pull-through with a short pouch are the best operative options.

RECOMMENDED READING

Vilanova-Sanchez A, Ivanov M, Halleran DR, Wagner A, Reck-Burneo CA, Ruth B, Fisher M, Ahmad H, Weaver L, Nash O, Buker D, Rentea RM, Hoover E, Maloof T, Wood RJ, Levitt MA. Total colonic Hirschsprung's disease: The hypermotility and skin rash protocol. *Eur J Pediatr Surg.* 2020 Aug; 30(4): 309–316.

DOI: 10.1201/9781003150015-14

MYTH: PULL-THROUGH FOR TCHD MUST BE AFTER POTTY-TRAINING AGE

Early is on time. On time is late. Late is unacceptable.

– Contributed by: Paul Waltz

TCHD patients who have undergone definitive pull-through, regardless of the age the pull-through is done, often have a high incidence of multiple stools and they usually develop a perineal rash. However, with the implementation of treatments before the pull-through to slow and thicken stools and a perineal skin protocol to treat the skin after the pull-through, symptoms can be minimized, even in patients who are not toilet trained. With implementation of this protocol, a pull-through in TCHD patients can be performed between the ages of 6 and 18 months.

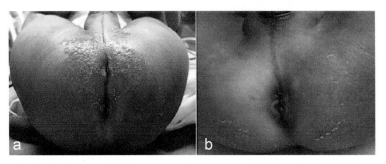

Figure 12.2 Perineal rash (a) 1 month following pull-through and (b) 3 months after skin care initiated in a child with TCHD.

Protocol for Treatment of Hypermotility

1. Skin care for perineal skin
   - Cyanoacrylate-based barrier liquid. Repeated every 2–3 days.
   - Proton pump inhibitors to reduce the acidity of stool.
   - Irrigations/saline small enemas (approximately 120 mL).
   - Water-soluble fiber (pectin).
2. Medical management for hypermotility
   - Loperamide if > 5 stools/day or > 30 mL/kg: 0.5–0.8 mg/kg divided daily (Imodium).
   - Cholestyramine max. 8 g divided daily.
   - Hyoscyamine (Levsin) – 0.125 mg tab/6 hours.
   - Diphenoxylate/atropine (Lomotil).
3. Monitor growth curve.
4. Monitor urine sodium (keep above 20 mmol/L).

ARE SODIUM LOSSES KEEPING MY CHRONIC STOMA PATIENTS FROM GAINING WEIGHT?

Ileostomies and, to a lesser extent, colostomies can lead to losses of sodium and bicarbonate. Sodium (Na^+) is needed to absorb glucose efficiently as the Na^+/glucose transporter does not work in the absence of sodium. Furthermore, with severe sodium depletion, aldosterone stimulates the absorption of most of the sodium filtered in the kidney, and this leaves limited sodium available for Na^+–H^+ ion exchange, leading to metabolic acidosis. A decrease in glucose absorption and metabolic acidosis can cause failure to thrive. The same amount of nutrition is not absorbed as well without sodium present in the lumen of the bowel.

Serial urine sodium checks are vital in all patients with a chronic ileostomy (or colostomy) and after an ileo-anal pull-through. If the urine sodium is less than 20 mmol/L, start sodium supplementation. To supplement sodium losses, the formula to keep in mind is to increase the sodium by 3 extra mEQ/kg/day and recheck in 1–2 months. The recipe for sodium supplementation is 1 teaspoon (5 mL) of salt plus 40 mL of water equals 2.5 mEQ

> The secret of getting ahead is getting started. The secret of getting started is breaking your complex overwhelming tasks into small manageable tasks, and then starting on the first one.
>
> **– Mark Twain**

of sodium per milliliter (mL). Once the urine sodium is corrected (to above 20 mmol/L), you should start to see improved weight gain. The improved weight gain is a result of better glucose absorption (enhanced by luminal sodium). Intravenous sodium supplementation will not correct the situation. In addition, the serum sodium can remain normal, despite a very low urine sodium. Thus, urine sodium provides better evidence of total body sodium depletion.

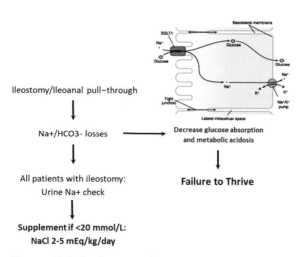

Figure 12.3 Sodium supplementation.

RECOMMENDED READING

O'Neil M, Teitelbaum DH. Total body sodium depletion and poor weight gain in children and young adults with an ileostomy: A case series. *Nutr Clin Pract.* 2014 Jun; 29(3): 397–401.

Schwarz KB. Sodium needs of infants and children with ileostomy. *J Pediatr.* 1983 Apr; 102(4): 509–513.

FAILURE TO THRIVE IN TOTAL COLONIC HIRSCHSPRUNG DISEASE

No amount of postoperative care undoes a bad operation.

– Contributed by: Marc Levitt

A 2-year-old girl with TCHD and an end ileostomy has been having trouble with weight gain. She is on G-tube feeds and presents with acute abdominal distension. The X-ray images are shown in Figure 12.4.

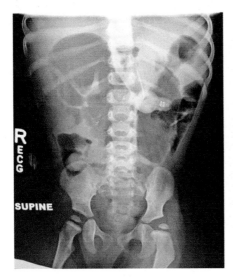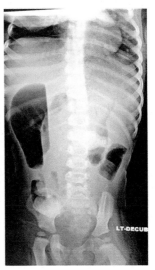

Figure 12.4 Distension noted on abdominal X-ray, but of what?

What do you think is going on? What is dilated?

In the X-rays shown in Figure 12.4, there is a dilated structure with an air fluid level, but it is not apparent what structure is distended. Possibilities include the small bowel or the defunctionalized colon. The most likely culprit for this patient's condition is a narrow stoma and thus dilated small bowel proximally, but do not forget about the defunctionalized colon. Air in that distal colon could be from bacterial overgrowth, which can lead to enterocolitis and even toxic megacolon.

What is your plan?

The patient did not improve on retrograde irrigations (via the stoma and via the rectum), and so she was taken to the operating room. The small bowel proximal to the stoma was very dilated, related to narrowing at the fascial level that was not detected on the initial exam. A biopsy of the ileostomy site showed the presence of ganglion cells. The stoma fascial site was revised. As the patient was known to have TCHD, a subtotal colectomy was performed, leaving the upper rectum as a Hartmann's pouch. With a better stoma and the colon removed, the patient thrived and was thus set up for a future pull-through.

CHAPTER 13

LATE DIAGNOSIS HIRSCHSPRUNG DISEASE

LATE DIAGNOSIS OF HIRSCHSPRUNG DISEASE

A 4-year-old boy with Down syndrome presents with severe constipation without a history of enterocolitis episodes. His contrast study is seen in Figure 13.1.

> Every stitch a masterpiece.
>
> **– Contributed by: Tarryn Gabler**

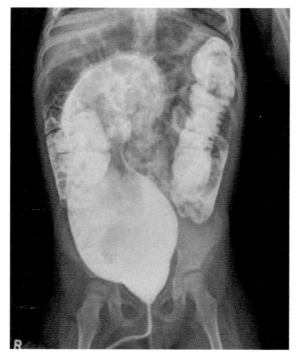

Figure 13.1 X-ray of patient with Down syndrome and severe constipation potentially due to underlying HD.

How would you proceed with diagnosing this patient?

HD is an important cause of constipation in a patient with Down syndrome. Anorectal manometry (AMAN) is a key first step to rule out that possibility.

- If there is an absent recto-anal inhibitory reflex (RAIR), then the patient needs a rectal biopsy. If the RAIR is absent and a rectal biopsy demonstrates no ganglion cells with hypertrophic nerves, then this is HD.
- If the biopsy shows ganglion cells but the RAIR is absent, then this could be internal sphincter achalasia, which would benefit from botulinum toxin injection of the anal sphincters.
- If the sphincters are normal and a RAIR is present, then no biopsy is needed. This represents functional constipation, which can be managed with laxatives, enemas, or antegrade flushes.

If this turns out to be HD, what would be your surgical plan?

If this patient has HD, management would be rectal irrigation for 1 or 2 months, then the surgeon can proceed with an HD pull-through (laparoscopy with biopsy plus transanal or transanal only). If irrigations are not tolerated or if the colon is massive, as it sometimes is in such a late diagnosis, the patient will need diversion with ileostomy or colostomy as a first step. In such an older child, when the transition zone is very low (rectal), a transanal-only approach done in prone position can be considered (Figure 13.2).

Think thrice, measure twice, cut once.

– **Contributed by: Martin Lacher**

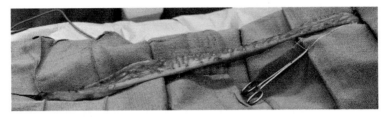

Figure 13.2 Pull-through of 45 cm of rectosigmoid, all done transanally.

A 14-YEAR-OLD WITH HIRSCHSPRUNG DISEASE

In a similar case, a 14-year-old boy with chronic distension and poor growth presents to your clinic. He has never had any episodes of enterocolitis. An AMAN shows an absent RAIR. A rectal biopsy shows no ganglion cells and hypertrophic nerves, confirming the diagnosis of HD (Figure 13.3).

> It's easier to stay out of trouble, than to get out of trouble.
>
> **– Fred Ryckman**

What would be your plan?

(a) Primary laparoscopic-assisted transanal pull-through.
(b) Leveling colostomy.
(c) Ileostomy with colonic biopsies and a future pull-through.
(d) Laxative therapy (with irrigations if needed).
(e) Irrigations for 3–4 months and then primary laparoscopic-assisted pull-through.
(f) Other.

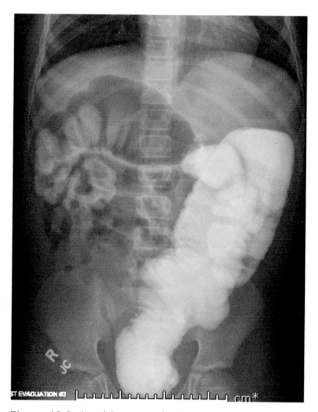

Figure 13.3 An older case of HD.

In this case, an ileostomy and colonic biopsies are best, to allow the colon to decompress; then plan a pull-through. Irrigations for several months could also be an option but might not be well-tolerated in an older patient.

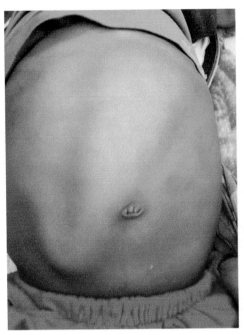 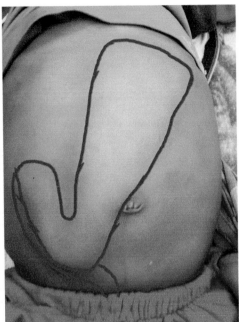

Figure 13.4

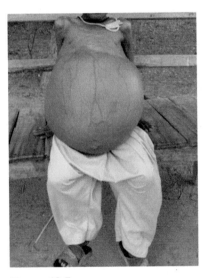 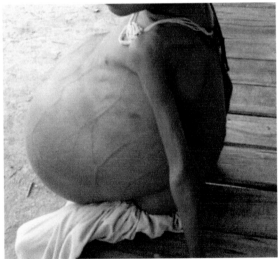

Figure 13.5

> I'm happy when everything we do in the OR works. I'm pretty unhappy if it fails. But we have to guard against being happy when the operation is *only* a technical success. The long haul is what counts.
>
> **– Thomas Starzl**

Shown in Figures 13.4 and 13.5 are some extreme examples of the abdominal exam in patients with a late diagnosis of HD. These situations are not uncommonly faced in the developing world. This type of HD is clearly phenotypically different from the expected presentation. Older HD diagnoses have chronic constipation, abdominal distention, and failure to thrive, and do not typically have enterocolitis.

Chapter 14

HIRSCHSPRUNG DISEASE MYTHS

MYTH: LAPAROSCOPIC SEROMUSCULAR BIOPSY ALONE CAN DETERMINE PULL-THROUGH LEVEL

Full-thickness biopsies give the pathologist more tissue (both plexuses) and decrease the chance that a transition zone will be missed. When the submucosal layer is not part of the sample and only the seromuscular layer is analyzed, there is a risk of missing nerve hypertrophy

> Sometimes the most conservative thing to do is a big operation.
>
> **– Michael Caty**

in the submucosal layer, a feature consistent with the transition zone. In the transition zone, large nerves often coexist with submucosal ganglia. Identification of multiple large nerves (e.g., more than two nerves >40 mm in one 400 field) is considered diagnostic of the transition zone and warrants additional surgery to get above the neuroanatomically abnormal bowel (Figure 14.1). This laparoscopic technique works well but only samples the seromuscular layer. If this technique is used to find the level, a confirmatory full thickness (all layers) biopsy is needed before sewing in the pull-through.

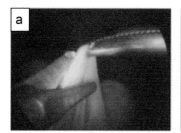 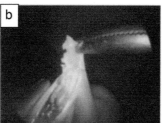 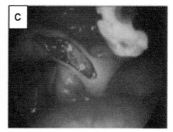

Figure 14.1 Laparoscopic seromuscular biopsy (a–c) utilizing laparoscopic scissors.

RECOMMENDED READING

Kapur RP. Histology of the transition zone in Hirschsprung disease. *Am J Surg Pathol*. 2016 Dec; 40(12): 1637–1646.

Smith C, Ambartsumyan L, Kapur RP. Surgery, surgical pathology, and postoperative management of patients with Hirschsprung disease. *Pediatr Dev Pathol*. 2020 Jan–Feb; 23(1): 23–39.

Veras LV, Arnold M, Avansino JR, Bove K, Cowles RA, Durham MM, Goldstein AM, Krishnan C, Langer JC, Levitt M, Monforte-Munoz H, Rabah R, Reyes-Mugica M, Rollins MD 2nd, Kapur RP, Gosain A, American Pediatric Surgical Association Hirschsprung Disease Interest Group. Guidelines for synoptic reporting of surgery and pathology in Hirschsprung disease. *J Pediatr Surg*. 2019 Oct; 54(10): 2017–2023.

PART III
FUNCTIONAL CONSTIPATION
AND FECAL INCONTINENCE

CHAPTER 15

BOWEL MANAGEMENT

BOWEL MANAGEMENT: HOW TO PREPARE A CHILD FOR THIS CARE

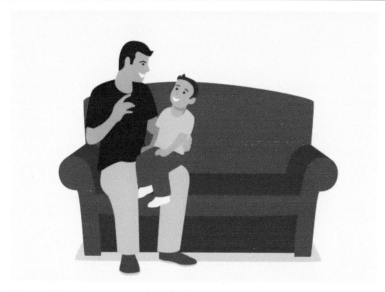

Figure 15.1 Preparing a child for bowel management.

The goal of bowel management is to find the right bowel routine for a child to clean out the colon every day. This means finding a system whereby the colon is made clean for 24 hours, with no passage of stool during the other hours, and without accidents or streaking in the under-wear. This regimen might include using medications (laxa-

> Children survive despite our medical interventions.
>
> **– Contributed by: Inbal Samuk**

tives), which provoke the colon to empty in a child who has the continence elements to control the stool. Or, it might mean an enema routine which mechanically empties the colon at a prescribed time. A bowel regimen has the potential to significantly improve a patient's quality of life by getting them out of diapers and allowing them to participate in school and extracurricular activities like a typical child. A tremendous positive change in self-esteem occurs once children are on a successful bowel regimen.

When talking to a child about bowel management, the parent should use words and sentences that the child can easily understand, while explaining that bowel management is a normal part of life. Using age-appropriate, empathetic, and positive words during the explanation of bowel management will show the child that this is a doable process. As soon as the child is able, they can be asked to gather supplies and partake in the process of the enema administration, as it allows them to take partial ownership and control over the process. Decreasing anxiety during enema administration will aid in the child looking forward to that designated time for enema administration and alleviate stress around that time. This can be done by saving a fun activity or favorite toy to play with that is reserved only for that time.

BOWEL MANAGEMENT FOR FECAL INCONTINENCE AND SOILING

When we least expect it, life sets us a challenge to test our courage and will-ingness to change; at such a moment, there is no point in pretending that nothing has happened or in saying that we are not yet ready. The challenge will not wait. Life does not look back.

– Paulo Coelho

Patients with a diagnosis of HD or an ARM who are not doing well with stooling after surgical repair will ben-efit from a Bowel Management Plan (BMP) to optimize medical management of their constipation or soiling. Likewise, those with fecal incontinence of a spinal or pelvic etiology (spina bifida, Sacrococcygeal teratoma) can also benefit. There are two main options for bowel management, either medical or mechanical treatment (Figure 15.2).

Medical management consists of treatment which targets modulation of hypomotility or hypermotil-ity. For patients with hypomotility, a good combination to start patients on is senna (a stimulant laxa-tive) and water-soluble fiber. This treatment is, of course, only applicable to patients with the anatomic capacity for voluntary bowel movements. For patients with hypermotility, a constipating diet and water-soluble fiber are needed to slow down motility and to achieve a one or two formed stool per day pattern of bowel movements. Sometimes loperamide needs to be added. If patients continue to struggle with hypermotility, small-volume enemas can be used to help keep patients clean. The mechanical treatment utilizes enemas, either performed retrograde through the anus or as antegrade flushes through a Malone appendicostomy. Flushes are composed of saline or water combined with an irritant such as glycerin or soap.

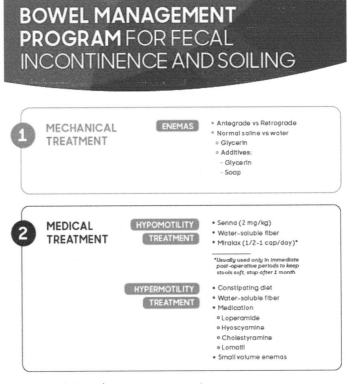

Figure 15.2 Bowel management options.

Chapter 16

EVALUATION OF CONSTIPATION AND SURGICAL ADJUNCTS

MANAGEMENT OF A PATIENT WITH FUNCTIONAL CONSTIPATION WITH FAILED MEDICAL MANAGEMENT

Patients with functional constipation can either be managed with medical management or surgical intervention. Medical management should start with optimizing laxative therapy or a trial of rectal enemas. For a patient with a long-standing history of functional constipation who has failed medical management (laxatives and/or rectal enemas), the physician should start with a contrast enema to evaluate for the degree of colonic dilation as well as any redundancy.

Five qualities for a learned and an expert surgeon – (1) Lady's finger (Gentle handling of tissues) – (2) Lion's heart (Boldness in decision making and prompt action) – (3) Eagle's eye (Watchfulness) – (4) Horse's legs (Stamina to stand) – (5) Camel's Belly (to carry out work without food and water).

– **Contributed by: Bu Nguyen**

The patient should then undergo an anorectal manometry (AMAN) to check for a recto-anal inhibitory reflex (RAIR), the resting pressures of the anal sphincters and for pelvic floor dyssynergia. If a RAIR is absent, then the patient should ideally get a rectal biopsy at the time of the AMAN to rule out HD. For an absent RAIR (if not HD) and for high resting pressure of the external sphincters, the patient should also be considered for an injection of botulinum toxin to treat internal sphincter achalasia or withholding. If the AMAN shows pelvic floor dyssynergia, the patient may also benefit from pelvic floor physiotherapy. Of note, AMAN results may be unreliable for patients who are very young (under one year of age) or those who cannot follow instructions during the AMAN. These patients may need a rectal biopsy and botulinum toxin injection into the anal canal done empirically without having AMAN data. Very often this treatment of the sphincters is what the patient needs, and they will then respond better to laxatives because their sphincters allow the rectum to empty.

For patients who have an intact RAIR or exhibit low resting pressures, neither a biopsy nor botulinum toxin is not needed. These patients should then proceed with an evaluation of colonic motility by colonic manometry (CMAN), sitzmark study, or nuclear scintigraphy. For surgical intervention, a Malone can be placed to provide a channel for antegrade flushes, with ongoing titration of the flush regimen on an individual basis. This option works in the vast majority of cases of constipation unresponsive to medical therapy and is also a great option for patients with behavioral limitations to achieving voluntary bowel movements. If the patient is successfully managed with flushes, after about 6–12 months, most patients can be transitioned to laxative therapy. If the flushes are unable to manage the patient's constipation, then, on very rare occasions, additional surgical intervention may be needed to resect the colon and remove any dysmotile segment as seen on the motility evaluation. Pelvic floor physiotherapy is a vital adjunct prior to considering a resection.

A vital investigation to troubleshoot ineffective flushes prior to considering surgical resection of the colon is assessment for reflux of the flush into the terminal ileum with a contrast study, as this is a possible cause of flush ineffectiveness or intolerance by the patient. The extent of resection, if one is needed, is guided by the colonic motility results, and options include a segmental sigmoid resection, if there is focal segmental dysfunction, extended colonic resection, if there is significant dilation or redundancy, or a total colonic resection if there is poor motility throughout the entire colon (Figure 16.1).

DOI: 10.1201/9781003150015-19

Why don't you try a different mistake?

– **Contributed by: Michael Phillips**

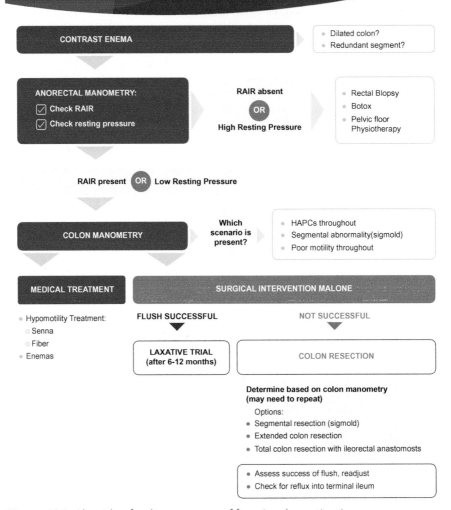

Figure 16.1 Algorithm for the treatment of functional constipation.

NINE-YEAR-OLD BOY WITH SEVERE CONSTIPATION

A 9-year-old boy presents to the clinic with severe constipation, daily cramping pain, and soiling. Multiple medical regimens have been tried, using laxatives and stool softeners, but with no improvement. Rectal enemas have also been tried, which have not worked. His plain X-ray and his contrast study are shown in Figure 16.2.

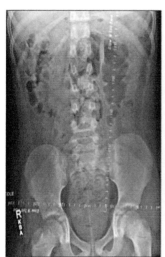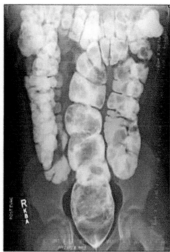

Figure 16.2 Scout film and contrast enema.

What would be your next diagnostic steps?
Would you perform a surgical intervention at this time?

From this description, we can conclude that he has failed medical management. Both medicines and enemas have not worked. So, we are now dealing with a more severe case of constipation with significant symptoms. For the next step, we need to do an AMAN. This study will show whether there is a RAIR, and, if present, this essentially rules out HD (Figure 16.3). If there is an absent RAIR, it is either HD (unlikely) or internal sphincter achalasia, and a rectal biopsy is needed as well as treatment with botulinum toxin. On occasion, you might find an older HD case that may have suffered for years with constipation and never had enterocolitis. If HD is ruled out, many times you can treat the sphincter first and avoid any surgical treatment (as this is an outlet problem not a colonic motility problem), and then reduce laxative use as soon as the sphincters perform more normally. Treatment of the sphincters is with botulinum toxin, which usually works and may need

Diagnosis	Hirschsprung Disease	Internal Sphincter Achalasia	Functional Constipation
AMAN results	Absent RAIR	Absent RAIR	Present RAIR
Biopsy results	Absent Ganglion cells Present hypertrophic nerves	Present Ganglion cells	Present Ganglion cells
Management	Pull-through	Botulinum toxin	CMAN, possible Malone or colon resection

Figure 16.3

to be repeated in 3–4 months. 100 units of botulinum toxin in 1-2 cc of saline is injected into the anal canal. Pelvic floor physiotherapy may also play a role.

What if the AMAN was normal? What would be your next diagnostic step? What surgical intervention, if any, would you offer?

In this case, if the sphincters are not contributing to the constipation, we need to assess colonic motility. Options include, in order of increasing accuracy, a sitzmark study, a radionuclide study, or a colonic manometry. You want to know which of the following three options you are dealing with:

1. Slow colonic motility, but activity throughout the colon.
2. Segmentally abnormal motility (usually the sigmoid).
3. Diffuse colonic dysmotility with no activity throughout the colon.

Motility Finding	Initial Treatment	Surgical Resection (if antegrade flushes fail)
Diffusely slow but HAPCs throughout	Malone	Sigmoid resection
Segmental dysmotility (sigmoid)	Malone	Sigmoid resection
Diffuse colonic dysmotility	Malone	Extended resection*

*For diffuse dysmotility cases, surgery entails a subtotal colectomy with ileorectal anastomosis, if balloon expulsion test is successful, and a Deloyers procedure with antegrade flushes, if the balloon expansion test fails. Pelvic floor physiotherapy should be done prior to this decision.

Figure 16.4

> We're not in this business to see what we can get away with.
>
> **– Siggie Ein, Contributed by: Jack Langer**

At this point, for all three scenarios, we should initially offer an antegrade flush option (Malone or cecostomy) (Figure 16.4). With antegrade flushes, the vast majority of patients will do well. For patients with slow motility, but with high amplitude propagated contractions (HAPCs) throughout the colon, this is a very reliable option. For the segmentally abnormal patient, antegrade flushes alone usually work (more than 90% of the time). For the diffusely dysmotile patient, flushes usually do not work (10% success). If antegrade flushes fail, then a resection may be required. However, pelvic floor physiotherapy should be done first as this is often the underlying problem.

Specific data and more precise numbers for each scenario are being developed through research done by the Pediatric Colorectal and Pelvic Learning Consortium (PCPLC; www.pcplc.org). These are relatively new ideas and emphasize the vital importance of collaboration with colleagues in GI/motility.

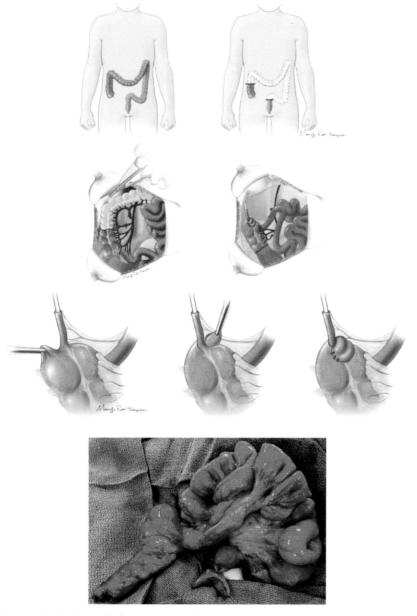

Figure 16.5 Extended resection (Deloyers procedure) plus Malone.

The Deloyers procedure for extended resection of the sigmoid, left, transverse, and part of the right colon plus Malone appendicostomy is illustrated in Figure 16.5. The right colon is anastomosed to the rectum and a Malone is placed in the lower quadrant. If the patient can empty their rectum (demonstrated by a successful balloon expulsion test), then a subtotal colectomy plus ileorectal anastomosis is the procedure of choice.

> If you are surrounded by seas, you are on an island. If you see only land, you are in-continent.
>
> **– Contributed by: Marc Levitt**

LIFELONG CONSTIPATION WITH BIOPSY SHOWING HYPERTROPHIC NERVES

You are judged by what you are willing to stop for.

– Fred Ryckman

A 9-year-old female presents to your clinic with lifelong constipation, a normal AMAN, and a present RAIR. She is on high-dose laxatives and has cramps and soiling. A rectal biopsy showed ganglion cells and hypertrophic nerves. Her contrast study is demonstrated in Figure 16.6.

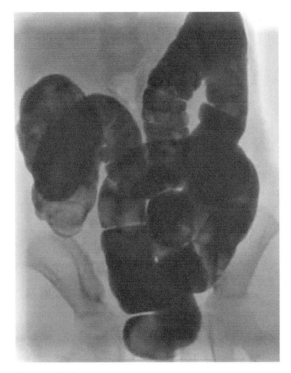

Figure 16.6

Can you exclude HD according to the AMAN biopsy results and the imaging? What would your treatment plan be?

HD can be excluded based on the normal AMAN results and present RAIR. With this information, the biopsy was not required. The presence of ganglion cells does confirm further that the patient does not have HD. Hypertrophic nerves are not necessarily related to HD; they can result from rectal dilation from poor emptying and long-standing constipation.

The contrast enema shows a redundant sigmoid and transverse colon. The clinical findings are most consistent with constipation that is refractory to medical management. As the current medical management was unsuccessful, and the sphincters are not the problem, the next step in management for this patient is a mechanical program: antegrade flushes through a Malone appendicostomy or rectal enemas. The vast majority of patients with functional constipation respond to mechanical flushes alone, without the need for colonic resection.

If a patient fails their mechanical regimen, only then should you consider colonic resection and that should be based on the motility evaluation and redundancy seen on contrast enema. In this unique case, both the sigmoid and transverse colon are redundant. Therefore, a resection of the sigmoid and left colon with an anastomosis between the transverse colon and the upper rectum is the best choice.

IS CONSTIPATION DUE TO HIRSCHSPRUNG DISEASE?

A 10-year-old boy presents to the clinic with severe constipation, unresponsive to a series of laxative regimens. He has daily cramping, poor appetite, and soiling. His contrast study is shown in Figure 16.7.

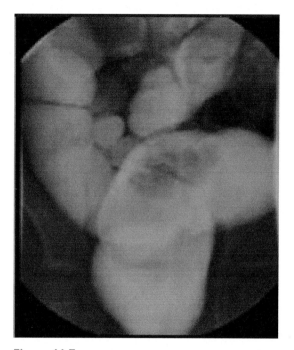

Figure 16.7

An awake AMAN was done, and the RAIR was absent. The rectal biopsy showed no ganglion cells in 100 levels. However, there was calretinin expression visible.

What would you do for this patient?

The possibilities include:
- (a) The patient has HD and needs a pull-through, but the biopsy should be repeated first.
- (b) The patient has internal sphincter achalasia and needs botulinum toxin, laxatives, and possibly a Malone.
- (c) The patient has functional constipation and just needs a Malone.
- (d) Although the patient does not have ganglion cells, calretinin presence means there are ganglion cells, excluding HD.

If there are no ganglion cells, does that mean HD? If there is no comment on hypertrophic nerves, then the answer is "no." A surgeon should not operate on a patient with *only* the absence of ganglion cells. You need more evidence. If there is calretinin expression, that means ganglion cells are nearby. If calretinin staining is positive, this is not a case of HD. More likely, this patient has internal sphincter achalasia, and the absence of ganglion cells is a sampling error related to dilation of the rectum. Therefore, botulinum toxin injection into the

And once the storm is over, you won't remember how you made it through, how you managed to survive. You won't even be sure whether the storm is really over. But one thing is certain. When you come out of the storm, you won't be the same person who walked in. That's what the storm's all about.

– Haruki Murakami

Tell me and I forget. Teach me and I remember. Involve me and I learn.

– Benjamin Franklin, Contributed by: Teresa Russell

anal sphincter, more laxative therapy, and a Malone for antegrade flushes are good treatment options. There is no need for a colostomy or an HD pull-through.

To confirm the results, the biopsy can be repeated. Also, this does not sound like an HD patient clinically, with no chronic distension, failure to thrive, or episode of enterocolitis. Severe chronic constipation alone is only rarely HD.

CHAPTER 17

MALONE APPENDICOSTOMY (ANTEGRADE) OR ENEMAS (RETROGRADE) FOR COLONIC CLEANING

UNDERSTANDING THE APPENDICEAL MESENTERY FOR MALONE CREATION

When performing the plication of the cecum around the appendix for a Malone appendicostomy, look closely at the appendiceal mesentery. There are two distinct anatomic vasculature patterns.

> Our eyes only see what our mind suspects.
>
> **– Alberto Peña**

For the case of mesentery with the appendiceal artery parallel to the appendix, see Figure 17.1.

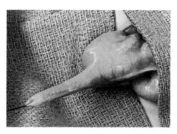 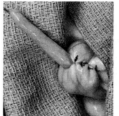 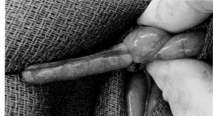

Figure 17.1 Appendiceal mesentery that parallels the appendix.

To create the plication, the appendix and mesentery are straightened, and the plication is created around the base of both.

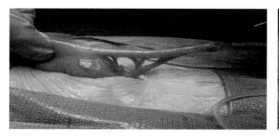 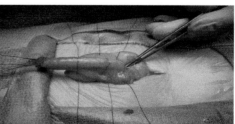

Figure 17.2 Appendiceal mesentery that is fenestrated.

For the case of mesentery with the appendiceal artery in a fenestrated pattern, see Figure 17.2.

A window is created between the perforating vessels in the mesentery, and the side of the cecum to be used for the wrap is pulled through each window to create the plication.

DOI: 10.1201/9781003150015-20

MALONE PLICATION – DO NOT OBSTRUCT THE TERMINAL ILEUM

When performing the plication of the cecum around the appendix, it is important to align the appendix so it does not kink the terminal ileum (Figures 17.3 and 17.4).

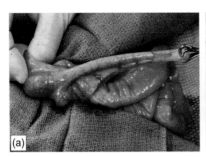 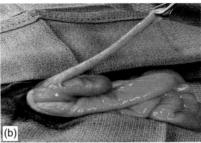

Figure 17.3 (a) Plication done toward the terminal ileum – wrong choice, (b) Plication done away from the terminal ileum – better choice.

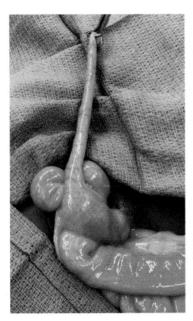 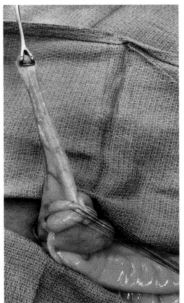

Figure 17.4 The plication, avoiding the terminal ileum.

NEO-MALONE

When a patient does not have an appendix, or the appendix needs to be used for other purposes (i.e. for a Mitrofanoff), a portion of the cecum or right colon can be tubularized to create a neo-Malone. A rectangle is marked on either side of a colonic vessel that runs transversely on both sides of the colon (Figure 17.5).

> In planning an operation, make sure that you are doing it for the right indication, and having decided the right indication, make sure that you do the right operation.
>
> **– Alastair Millar**

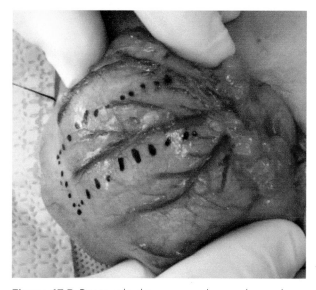

Figure 17.5 Rectangle drawn around a cecal vessel.

Then, this flap is lifted (Figure 17.6).

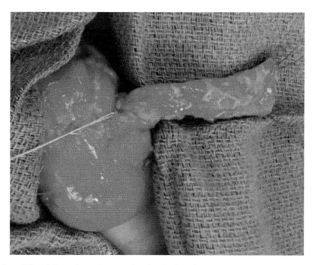

Figure 17.6 Cecal flap lifted for the planned tubularization.

Keep in mind the direction of the tubularized flap. Once the flap is tubularized (Figure 17.7), it needs to be laid back on the colon for the plication so the orifice of the newly created tube faces the location where the abdominal wall orifice will be created. This is either the umbilicus or the right lower quadrant.

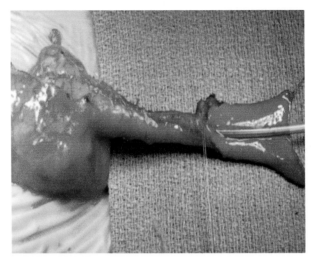

Figure 17.7 Tubularization of cecal flap.

CIRCULAR ANASTOMOSIS FOR MALONE

Always bring a gun to a knife fight.

– **Michael Caty**

One option for the umbilical anastomosis in a Malone appendicostomy is a circular anastomosis at the base of the umbilicus. This is a very reproducible technique and is ideal when there is another incision already on the abdomen which can be used for the cecal plication. Evert the umbilicus, cut a circle in the umbilical skin, and then suture the circle of the cut appendix to the circle made in the skin. The umbilicus can be reduced to create a hidden orifice (Figure 17.8).

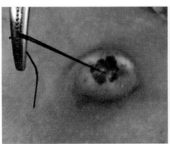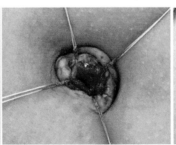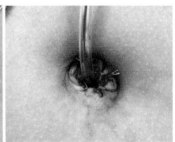

Figure 17.8 Circular appendix to umbilical skin anastomosis.

MALONE – Y–V ANASTOMOSIS

Another option for the umbilical anastomosis in a Malone appendicostomy is a Y–V anastomosis that creates a triangular flap that covers the opening, allowing the umbilicus to appear more natural. This is the preferable technique during a laparoscopic Malone, as the umbilical fascia can be incised and the cecum delivered extracorporeally to perform the plication, but no infraumbilical skin incision is needed.

Each step of the Y–V appendix to umbilical skin anastomosis is shown in Figure 17.9 and the steps are numbered as follows:

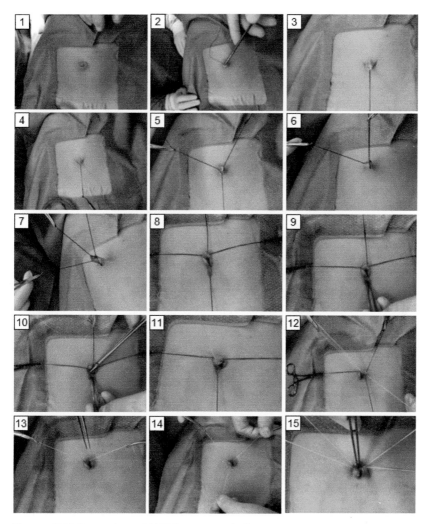

Figure 17.9 Procedure of Y–V Anastomosis Steps.

1. Umbilicus
2. Suture at bottom of V
3. V on stretch
4. V now marked
5. Cutting of the V
6. Extension to a Y
7. Cutting of the V and Y
8. V now mobile
9. V ready for anastomosis to appendix
10–14. Sewing of V–V
    15. V–V complete, stem of Y ready to be closed

MALONE FINISHING TOUCHES: SMALL DETAILS TO AVOID COMPLICATIONS

The goal is not at the end of the road. The road IS the goal.

– Contributed by: Matt Ralls

Following a Malone appendicostomy, a feeding tube or Foley catheter is left across the appendiceal–umbilical anastomosis (Figure 17.10). The tube is left in place for 1 month, but it is used within a day or two following surgery (after the resumption of a regular diet) for the daily antegrade flushes.

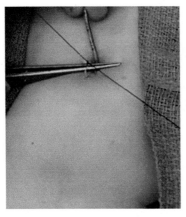
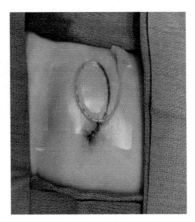

Figure 17.10 Tube left in umbilicus.

After 1 month, the family is taught how to use the Malone by catheterizing the tract. A Coudé catheter is easiest, because the stiffness and angle of the tip makes it easier to pass through the tract without injury (Figure 17.11).

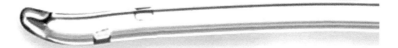

Figure 17.11 Coudé catheter.

At this clinic visit, the family should be provided with a silicone stopper or alternative. A simple clear plastic dressing can be used to keep it in place (Figure 17.12). The ACE stopper is left in place for 6 months to mature the tract and thereby avoid early stenosis. An indwelling balloon device, like those used for a gastrostomy tube, is another option. Alternatively, the patient can pass the tube a second time each day to keep the tract patent.

Science is made up of mistakes, but they are mistakes which are useful to make, because they lead little by little to the truth.

– Contributed by: Luca Giacomello

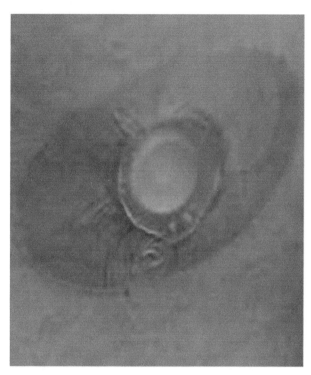

Figure 17.12 Malone site stopper in place and taped down.

ACE STOPPER SUBSTITUTION

> When you have made a mistake and you want to walk away from a situation, that is when you need to lean in.
>
> **– Contributed by: Katie Worst**

Antegrade continence enemas (ACEs) can be performed through a Malone appendicostomy, cecal flap neoappendix, or a tube cecostomy. When utilizing a tissue conduit such as a Malone or a cecal flap neoappendix, a stopper may be utilized to prevent leakage of gas and stool and act as a stent to prevent stricturing of the enterocutaneous anastomosis. A silicone ACE stopper can be substituted with a soft 8 Fr nasogastric tube that has been cut to length with two or three knots tied in the top or a cut and knotted Coudé catheter (Figure 17.13).

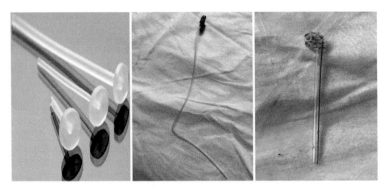

Figure 17.13 Options for the ACE orifice.

CHAPTER 18

MALONE COMPLICATIONS AND TROUBLESHOOTING

MALONE PROLAPSE

Sometimes a Malone appendicostomy can prolapse, usually owing to the opening in the fascia being too large. An easy fix for this is to mobilize the distal Malone, resect the prolapsed portion, and make the fascial opening tighter, incorporating the serosa of the appendix to prevent future prolapse.

The images seen in Figure 18.1 show the repair of a Malone prolapse. The pictures in the top row, from left to right, show the mobilization of the excess mucosa, placement of circumferential sutures around the excess mucosa, and mobilization of the appendix. The pictures in the bottom row, from left to right, show the trimming of excess appendiceal mucosa, the new circular appendix to umbilical skin anastomosis, and the completed anastomosis.

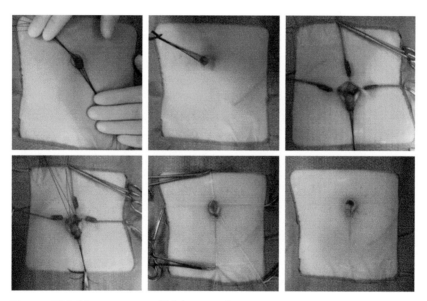

Figure 18.1 Management of Malone prolapse.

DOI: 10.1201/9781003150015-21

THE ACE STOPPER OR CATHETER IS STUCK. WHAT DO I DO?

The absence of options clears the mind.

– Craig Lillehei

This question is common in the colorectal world. After surgery, families go home and go about their normal flush routine. Everything is going according to plan, and the ACE stopper or catheter has suddenly become stuck. The family reaches out in a panic for help, wondering if this is normal and has ever happened to anyone else. Yes, we reassure them, this problem is common. Somehow, the stopper or catheter gets tied in a knot inside the patient. Instruct the family to cut off the round part of the ACE stopper or the catheter outside of the patient, and then advise them to advance a Coudé catheter with lubrication through the antegrade channel just like they would normally do as part of the flush routine. Reassure the family that the tiny silicone piece from the ACE stopper or end of the catheter will not cause any harm and will come out in the stool with the next flush.

THE ANTEGRADE OR RECTAL ENEMA IS NOT WORKING

If a rectal enema regimen does not seem to be working well or as anticipated, always make sure to obtain a contrast study via the Malone or cecostomy to evaluate the patient's anatomy and simulate the flush using contrast (Figure 18.2). Be aware of the possibility of a stricture at a previous colostomy closure site, which could impede the effectiveness of the enema and will become apparent on the study if it is present. Surgical intervention will be required to resect the strictured colon to correct the problem.

> You can't unscrew something by screwing it more.
>
> **– AR Moossa, Contributed by: Julia Grabowski**

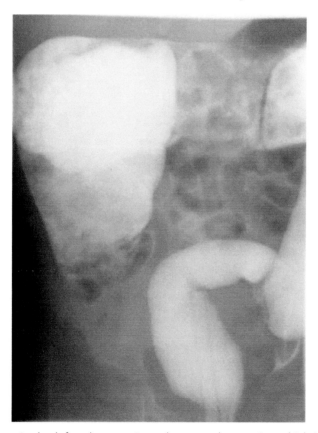

Figure 18.2 Stricture in the left colon at prior colostomy closure site, which impeded the antegrade flush.

A KEY STEP TO TROUBLE-SHOOTING ANTEGRADE FLUSH ISSUES

A knot that's not neat need not be knotted.

**– Dr Christopher Bartels,
Contributed by: Paul Waltz**

When a patient is experiencing difficulty performing daily antegrade flushes via a Malone or cecostomy, it is important to investigate the effectiveness of the flush. A contrast study done through the Malone or cecostomy can "mimic" the flush and show you the course of the flush.

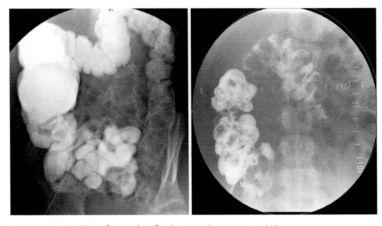

Figure 18.3 Flow from the flush into the terminal ileum.

Be aware that the flush can reflux into the terminal ileum in some patients, instead of flowing through the large intestine (Figure 18.3). As a result, the flush will not work well for these patients, and they will often experience side effects of nausea and abdominal discomfort. Of course, a large volume of the flush does not therefore enter the colon, so the flush is ineffective. The problem, if identified, can be resolved by placing a longer catheter into the Malone, which will direct the flush to the colon. This is a procedure performed by interventional radiology. Or, if the patient is cathing the Malone, they should put the catheter in deeper. Correct passage of the catheter into the deep right colon can be confirmed in the radiology suite.

URINARY RETENTION CAUSING OBSTRUCTION

A 17-year-old female with functional constipation had a motility evaluation which showed diffuse colonic dysmotility. There was an intact RAIR and no HAPCs on colonic manometry anywhere in her colon. On her AMAN, she passed the balloon explusion test (BET). Despite multiple treatment attempts, including with laxatives and enemas, her condition did not improve. Thus, a subtotal colectomy with an ileorectal anastomosis was performed. The patient did well at first, but, 3 months later, she came to the emergency department with impressive abdominal distension. The initial abdominal radiograph is shown in Figure 18.4.

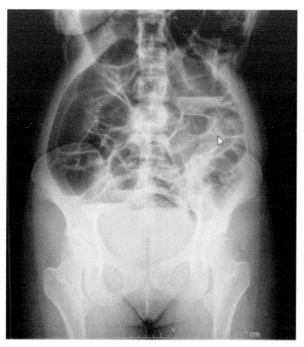

Figure 18.4 Small bowel distension and a pelvic mass lucency in the pelvis.

What is the cause of the patient's condition? What treatment does this patient need?

To exclude an anastomotic problem, a contrast enema was performed, which demonstrated a patent anastomosis without stenosis. The cause of the problem lies in a large pelvic mass that can be seen on the X-ray. This was in fact the bladder, which was massively distended, and the patient was in urinary retention. With drainage of the bladder, her symptoms markedly improved. Thereafter, with timed voiding, this problem did not recur.

CONTINUED CONSTIPATION DESPITE ANTEGRADE OR RETROGRADE ENEMAS

A passing mark in surgery is 100%.

– Bernie Langer, hepatobiliary surgeon and father of Jack Langer

Retrograde or antegrade enemas are effective treatment options for constipation management. Generally, it is not recommended to use oral medications along with these enemas, as it changes the predictability of the enema output. Some patients with poor colonic motility or severe constipation will experience continued difficulty and/or pain when trying to pass the enema solution, despite optimization of the enema solution (Figure 18.5). When this occurs, it is helpful to add ½–1 capful of polyethylene glycol (PEG) 3350 PO daily to soften the stool. The adjustment makes it easier to evacuate the enema solution/stool and often increases the effectiveness of the flush. It is necessary to titrate the PEG 3350 dose as needed for effect. Additionally, the timing to give this medicine is key to avoid leakage prior to the enema time.

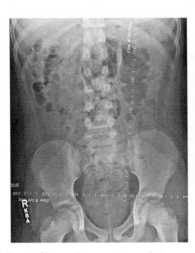 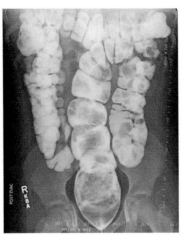

Figure 18.5 Scout film and contrast study in a patient with severe constipation.

RIGHT COLON STOOL ACCUMULATION

A 9-year-old female with a cloacal malformation and Malone appendicostomy for 6 years presents to clinic. Her flush regimen is 400 mL normal saline (NS) + 30 mL glycerin + 30 mL Castille soap, which the family reports works well, but the patient has occasional nighttime soiling and vomiting when enemas are not productive. A

> Out beyond ideas of wrongdoing and rightdoing there is a field. I'll meet you there.
>
> **– Rumi**

review of her contrast enema and an abdominal X-ray revealed a dilated right colon with a large stool burden (Figure 18.6).

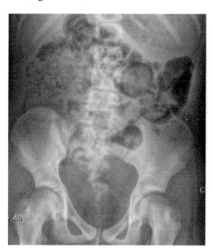 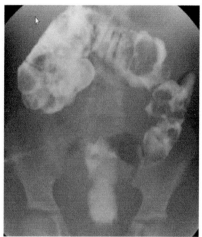

Figure 18.6

The following change is made to the flush directions to try to empty the right colon: concentrate the flush to 100 mL NS + 30 mL glycerin + 30 mL Castille, administer, and have the patient lie on the right side for 10–20 minutes, followed by administration of the remaining 300 mL NS volume.

The parents report nausea, cramping, and sweating with the initial regimen. The flush is adjusted again to an initial flush of 200 mL NS + 30 mL glycerin + 30 mL Castille, followed by 200 mL normal saline. The family then reports improved stool output and only an occasional small smear in the pull-up. An abdominal X-ray 1 month later revealed no stool accumulation (Figure 18.7).

The key to this bowel management was liquifying the stool in the right colon with a low volume concentrated flush lying the patient on their right side, and then flushing through with saline.

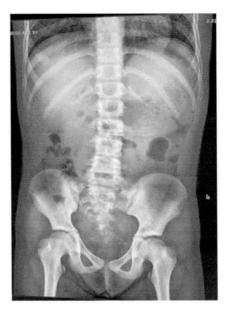

Figure 18.7 Follow-up X-ray with new flush regimen.

Records are always made to be broken, no matter what they are. Anybody can do anything that they set their mind to.

– Michael Phelps

Patients who have been on antegrade flushes for several years can, for reasons not quite understood, develop dilation and stool accumulation in the right colon that interferes with the effectiveness of the flush. This can be addressed with the previously described strategy.

MIDLINE CECUM

In this case, notice that the cecum is in the midline, which may occur from time to time. You must keep this anatomic fact in mind as you care for this patient, as a stool in the cecum on a plain abdominal X-ray might be misinterpreted as stool in the rectosigmoid. You may be successfully cleaning the rectum and sigmoid but not realize it, because stool in the cecum is incorrectly thought to be stool in the rectosigmoid (Figure 18.8).

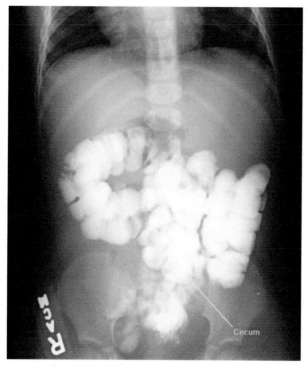

Figure 18.8

IS THE ANTEGRADE FLUSH COCKTAIL TOO STRONG?

Bad plan, executed poorly.

– Fred Ryckman

When a patient reports new-onset soiling between antegrade flushes after a period of cleanliness following a Malone procedure, the efficacy of the flush should be assessed with an abdominal X-ray. It is important to be aware that as the colon becomes accustomed to the antegrade flushes in the months following implementation, the enema recipe may need to be adjusted to prevent overstimulation by the enema itself. If a patient is reporting new-onset soiling and the X-ray reveals no stool accumulation, the amount of irritant should be decreased (Figure 18.9).

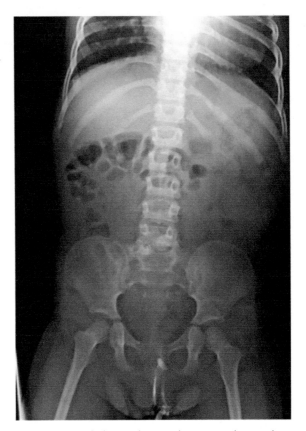

Figure 18.9 Abdominal X-ray showing a clean colon.

For example, an antegrade flush of 500 mL saline + 30 mL glycerin might be overstimulating the colon. Reduce the cocktail to 500 mL saline + 20 mL glycerin. Symptoms and an X-ray should be reassessed 3–5 days after the change to ensure that no further modifications are warranted.

INCREASING PATIENT COMFORT WITH RECTAL ENEMA ADMINISTRATION

Patients receiving daily rectal enemas typically have a minimum dwell time of 10 minutes. Many children find it challenging to sit still for this length of time, and complicating the administration is the cumbersome gravity bag attached to the Foley catheter. It must remain at a greater height than the child, often "tethering" the child to an area.

Utilizing a Kelly clamp to seal off the Foley catheter allows the child to separate from the gravity bag and move around (Figures 18.10–18.12). This allows for more comfortable positioning of the child during the dwell time, leading to greater compliance with the enema administration. In addition, the plastic Kelly clamp does not damage the tubing as a metal hemostat would, making it able to be connected and disconnected multiple times when parents are reusing the Foley catheter.

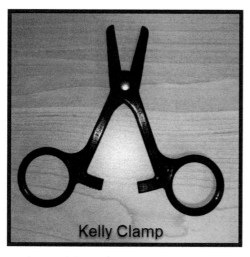

Figure 18.10 Kelly clamp used to seal the catheter.

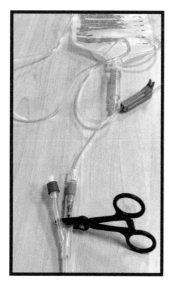

Figure 18.11 Kelly clamp on the tubing.

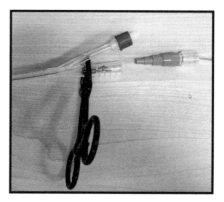

Figure 18.12 Another view of the Kelly clamp on the tubing.

LARGE-VOLUME ENEMA TROUBLESHOOTING

> We didn't lose. We just ran out of time.
>
> **– Vince Lombardi**

Large-volume enemas are an effective BMP for many children with fecal incontinence. However, it may take the child a few days to get acclimated to the administration. Two common issues when delivering a high-volume rectal enema include:

1. Abdominal discomfort upon instillation.
   - How to solve this problem:
     - ○ Slow the infusion.
       - ■ Typically, instructions are to instill over 5–10 minutes. However, when first beginning the enemas, the parent may need to slow this down to closer to 15 minutes.
     - ○ Warm the solution.
       - ■ Most base solutions are room temperature, which is much cooler than the average body temperature. This temperature change can lead to cramping. Warming the solution beforehand in conjunction with slowing it down can help with this discomfort.
       - ■ Note: <u>Warming should never be done in a microwave</u>. Instead, place the solution in a gravity bag or graduated cylinder and place it in a large bowl of very hot water to warm. This method is also commonly used when warming a baby bottle.

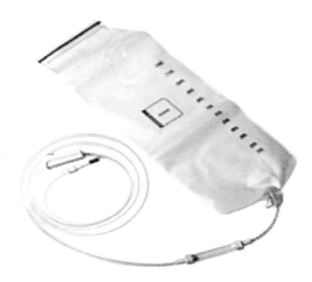

Figure 18.13 Enema bag and tubing.

2. Leaking of enema fluid around the catheter.
   - How to solve this problem:
     - ○ Double-check balloon inflation.

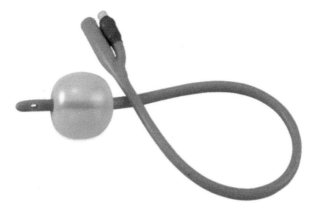

Figure 18.14 Foley catheter with balloon inflated.

- ■ The balloon at the end of the catheter should be checked for any manufacturer defects and to verify that it maintains the air or water placed inside. Typically, 10–20 mL of air or water is enough to create a seal; however, depending on the patient's anorectal anatomy, a larger catheter, with a larger balloon (up to 90 mL), may need to be utilized.

> So often in life, things that you regard as an impediment turn out to be great, good fortune.
>
> **– Ruth Bader Ginsburg**

- ○ Create tension.
  - ■ Once the catheter has been inserted and the balloon inflated, a constant and steady pressure must be held on the end of the catheter by pulling back to provide tension to create a seal and decrease leaking.

OPTIONS FOR INDEPENDENCE WITH BOWEL MANAGEMENT

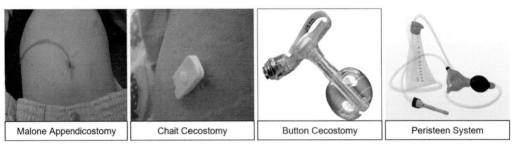

| Malone Appendicostomy | Chait Cecostomy | Button Cecostomy | Peristeen System |

Figure 18.15 Options for colonic flushes.

Surgical (Antegrade) Options

Catheterization via Malone appendicostomy: Pass a catheter through a channel in the appendix to access the colon. The opening is hidden in the belly button or right lower quadrant. This option offers independence in older children, allowing them to perform flushes while sitting on the toilet. It requires the ability to sit on the toilet for 1 hour. A Malone can be combined with a Mitrofanoff procedure for intermittent urinary catheterizing. If the appendix is unavailable, a neo-Malone procedure can be performed. Potential complications include stricture, prolapse, infection, false channel, and leakage.

Chait tube via Malone or cecostomy: Skin level device for flushes. This tube offers independence in older children to perform flushes while sitting on the toilet. They need to connect tubing to the device. It requires the ability to sit on the toilet for 1 hour and requires tube changes in interventional radiology (families cannot change the tube at home). Similar potential complications as for a G-tube exist, including granulation tissue, leakage, and infection. Also, the tube can fall out and need to be replaced.

Button device in the Malone or cecostomy: Skin level device for flushes. This type of tube offers independence in older children to perform flushes while sitting on the toilet. They need to connect tubing to the device. It requires the ability to sit on the toilet for 1 hour. It has the advantage of a balloon which holds the device in place and reduces leakage. Families can be taught to change the tube at home. Similar potential complications exist for a G-tube, including granulation tissue, leakage, and infection. Also, the tube can fall out and need to be replaced. The button device is sometimes not covered by insurance.

Non-Surgical (Retrograde) Option

Peristeen system: Offers independence in older children to perform flushes while sitting on the toilet. This option uses single-use pre-lubricated rectal catheters, utilizing tap water for flushes. Sit time on the toilet is reduced to 20–40 minutes, because it relies on a pump mechanism and air pressure rather than gravity flow. The enema system is expensive, insurance approval is often difficult, and trained providers need to teach the family how to use the product. It may not be as effective for bowel cleanout as the gravity method with foley balloon as described earlier (may need to add stimulants and/or stool softener, which are not easily added to the peristeen system).

HYDRO-ULTRASOUND TO ASSIST WITH BOWEL IRRIGATION

To optimize bowel management, an interesting option is to use hydro-ultrasound. The bowel irrigation can be done while doing an abdominal ultrasound. With this technique, you can see how much stool is in the bowel and what volume is required to disimpact and flush the

Trust no one except your mother, and keep a close eye on her.

– Contributed by: Marcus Jarboe

bowel properly. Figure 18.16 shows the fluid-filled rectum with some stool fragments inside on the right, and the sigmoid filled with stool, and some fluid reaching this loop on the left.

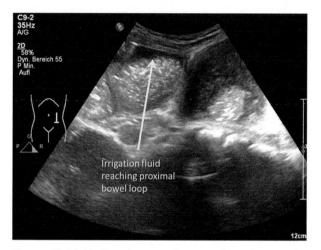

Figure 18.16 Hydro-ultrasound to assist bowel irrigation.

PROPER METHOD FOR RECTAL ENEMA ADMINISTRATION

When teaching parents to give rectal enemas to their child, instruct them to follow the steps shown below (Figure 18.17):

Proper Method for Rectal Enema Administration

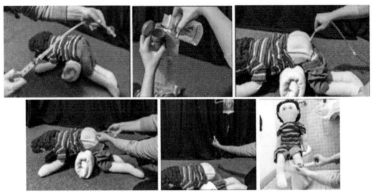

Figure 18.17 Enema technique.

1. Test the balloon on the catheter to ensure there is no leak.
   - Pull back the syringe plunger to fill it with 10–20 mL of air, then screw it onto the small port of the catheter and push the plunger in, filling the balloon with air. If the balloon does not inflate, do not use the catheter. Pull the plunger back to withdraw the air out of the balloon. Make sure the balloon is completely deflated before removing the syringe from the port.
2. Mix the prescribed enema recipe.
   - Mix the prescribed amount of normal saline and additives in a measuring container to ensure exact measurements. Then roll the clamp on the tubing of the gravity bag down to pinch off or "clamp" the tube closed before pouring the normal saline and additives into the gravity bag. Mix gently by tilting the bag back and forth, then hang the bag on a hook or shower rod. Squeeze the drip chamber hard to fill it partway with liquid, then open the clamp by rolling it up; allow fluid to run through the tubing until it drips out the end, then close the clamp (roll it back down).
3. Insert the catheter.
   - Position the child on their knees with buttocks up, a rolled towel under their abdomen, and their head resting on a pillow. This will let the parents see what they are doing. Once the parents are comfortable giving the enemas, the child may lie on their side if they prefer that position.
   - Lubricate the catheter by dipping it in a water-soluble lubricating jelly, then insert it about 4–6 inches into the rectum, and then screw the syringe gently onto the small port of the catheter. Gently inflate the balloon by pushing down on the syringe plunger. *While holding the plunger down,* unscrew and remove the syringe.
4. Give the enema.
   - Pull back very gently on the catheter until you meet resistance. This pulls the balloon against the inside of the anus to provide a seal and helps prevent leaks. Connect the tubing of the gravity bag to the large port on the catheter. Push it in tightly so it does

not leak. Open the roller clamp on the enema bag, and let the enema drip in over 5–10 minutes. Closing the roller clamp partway or lowering the height of the hanging bag will slow down the flow. Close the roller clamp when the

enema has all gone in. If the enema liquid leaks out of the child, either the catheter is not sealed to the rectum well (pull back a little more), or the balloon is not inflated enough (add more air next time).

5. Hold the enema inside.
   - For the enema to work the best, the child must *hold the enema solution in their rectum for 10 minutes* after it is all inside. It is normal for the child to complain of fullness or cramping during the "holding" time. The soapy water is irritating the child's colon to induce the colon to empty stool.
   - If the child has a lot of pain or vomits, slow down the enema or warm it up by sitting the enema bag in a bowl of warm water before you give it. **Never** microwave an enema!
6. Move the child to the toilet.
7. Remove the catheter.
   - Attach the syringe to the small catheter port and pull back on the plunger. This will remove the air and deflate the balloon. Allow the catheter to slip out of the bottom. The enema liquid and stool will also begin to come out.
8. Sit on the toilet.
   - Have the child sit on the toilet for approximately 40 minutes to let all of the stool and enema liquid come out. If the child has accidents in the 1–2 hours after the enema, they probably did not sit long enough.
   - For young children who have trouble sitting still, have them get up after 20 minutes and wash their face/brush their teeth, then sit back down for the rest of the time. Do not have them leave the bathroom!
9. Clean up.
   - Rinse the bag with soapy water and hang to dry. Flush the catheter with soapy water using the 60 mL syringe.

PROPER POSITIONING FOR EFFECTIVE ELIMINATION

I have never regretted doing an exploratory laparotomy for a patient I was worried about, but I certainly have said, "I should have been here 24 hours earlier."

– Marc Levitt

For any patient struggling with constipation or fecal incontinence, one of the first things to assess is the patient's position when they are trying to have a bowel movement. Posture and position can have a significant impact on the muscles of the pelvic floor, which are responsible for both keeping stool and urine in and letting them out. When sitting on the toilet, the ideal position is to sit with the knees hip-width apart and slightly higher than the hips, with the feet elevated on a stool, and to lean slightly forward with the elbows on the knees (Figure 18.18). This position allows the muscle that typically keeps the rectum "kinked off" to relax, allowing the rectum to straighten and empty completely. The other muscles of the pelvic floor relax as well.

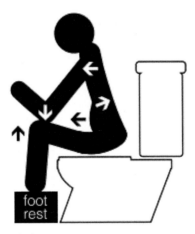

Figure 18.18 Positioning for stool elimination.

Proper breathing can also help relax the pelvic floor. Breathing using the diaphragm, which is a muscle higher up in the abdomen, is very useful. Patients can practice diaphragmatic breathing by placing a hand over their belly and breathing in a way that causes their belly to rise while breathing in and fall while breathing out. Some patients may have a tough time relaxing their pelvic floor muscles and coordinating their breathing in a way that allows them to have effective bowel movements.

A referral to pelvic floor physiotherapy can be made for patients who have difficulty relaxing their pelvic floor muscles. Pelvic floor therapists are physical therapists specifically trained in the pelvic floor muscles and many common bowel and bladder issues. They can help patients strengthen and relax those muscles while also helping them coordinate their breathing and pushing to have more comfortable and complete bowel movements.

WHAT TO DO WHEN YOU CANNOT INSERT THE CATHETER INTO THE MALONE ORIFICE

The inability to insert a catheter into the Malone orifice is a common problem for patients. The following steps are recommended to aid in catheter insertion:

> Under promise, over deliver.
>
> **– Tom Peters**

1. Ensure that a sufficient amount of water-soluble lubricant is applied to the catheter every time it is inserted into the Malone channel. This will help to guide the catheter in and eliminate any resistance.
2. Provide a relaxing and calming environment. A crying and screaming child will have a tense abdomen, which can make catheter insertion very difficult.
3. Have the patient lie down flat and take a few deep breaths. When inserting the catheter, slightly rotate or spin the catheter as you advance it into the channel. Make sure that the curved tip (Coudé) is pointing downward when initially entering the channel (Figure 18.19).

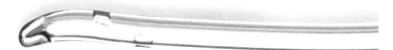

Figure 18.19 Curved tip of the Coudé catheter pointed down for insertion into channel.

4. Draw a warm bath and allow the patient to soak in the tub for 20 minutes. The warm water should help to soften the tissue. Repeat steps 1–3. A warm bath soak of the Malone orifice helps in many cases. If a warm bath is not an option, you can instead place a warm, moist washcloth over the Malone site for 20 minutes.

If the patient or family still cannot advance the catheter after these steps, they should not force the catheter. The healthcare team will be needed to rescue the tract. Usually this requires the help of interventional radiology.

A PATIENT WITH A SPINAL CORD ANOMALY AND SOILING

Three decades of learning for a surgeon: first how to operate, second when to operate, third when not to operate.

– Contributed by: Rambha Rai

Bowel management needs for children with spina bifida or spinal dysraphism depend on the patient's age and lesion level (Figure 18.20). It is also important to identify any other parameters affecting the bowels such as family willingness, physical barriers to care, school situation, and ambulatory status.

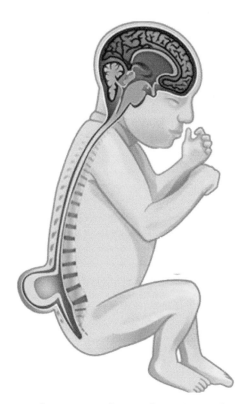

Figure 18.20 Artistic drawing of a patient with a myelomeningocele.

There are multiple options for bowel management, including stool softeners, suppositories, retrograde enemas, stimulant laxatives, and antegrade flushes. The key first determinant is to assess the patient's capacity for voluntary bowel movements. Often, urinary control is an excellent predictor of potential bowel control.

Many such patients have the capacity for bowel control and voluntary bowel movements. For those without this potential, or to help them realize this potential, a mechanical emptying program (retrograde enemas or antegrade flushes) is beneficial.

LOW-VOLUME ENEMAS FOR HYPERMOTILITY

Typically, patients with hypermotility are treated with a constipating diet, water-soluble fiber supplementation, and loperamide. Even with these medications, many patients continue to have frequent bowel movements, particularly while sleeping, and this can lead to diaper rash. Once you get to this point in the "hypermotility pathway", it is recommended to start patients on medica-

> Courage does not always roar. Sometimes courage is the quiet voice at the end of the day saying, '*I will try again tomorrow*'.
>
> **– Mary Anne Radmacher**

tions that have a significant side effect profile. Just prior to this, a safe and effective alternative is to do a small-volume enema of 150–250 mL NS + 10–20 mL glycerin at bedtime. This often eliminates overnight stooling for the patient and minimizes the number of bowel movements they have the next day, sometimes negating the need for additional medications. This low-volume enema can easily be administered using an empty enema bottle filled with the above contents. Evidence of hypermotility is a completely empty colon in a patient passing multiple stools daily, as shown in Figure 18.21.

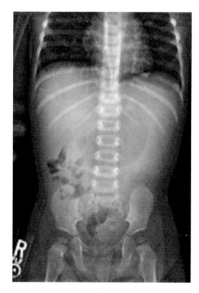

Figure 18.21 X-ray shows a completely clean colon, consistent with hypermotility.

SEVERE PERINEAL RASH

An 18-month-old boy with a history of HD has severe skin excoriation. He is 6 months post-ileoanal pull-through for TCHD done at another institution. His exam findings are shown in Figure 18.22.

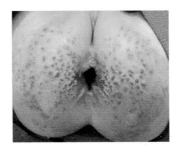

Figure 18.22 Perineum of this patient.

How would you manage this patient? Which options below would you do?
- (a)   A constipating diet with loperamide and water-soluble fiber.
- (b)   Daily enemas.
- (c)   Skincare only.
- (d)   Diverting stoma.
- (e)   Additional medical treatments for hypermotility (e.g., hyoscyamine (Levsin), cholestyramine).

The anus is patulous and the skin is severely excoriated from constant stooling. In this case, the sphincters and/or dentate line may have been damaged at the time of his operation. This patient needs an EUA with an assessment of the dentate line and sphincters. A trial of a strict constipating diet, plus bulking fiber and loperamide, is a reasonable start to slow and thicken the bowel movements. More aggressive agents to combat hypermotility, such as hyoscyamine and cholestyramine, may also improve the situation. A daily enema regimen is very helpful to mechanically evacuate the bowel and prevent continuous leakage of stool. Reducing stool contact with skin and meticulous skin care are required to heal the skin breakdown. An ileostomy might be needed here to control his symptoms. A new idea in such desperate situations is to tighten up the sphincters surgically.

Many patients develop severe skin breakdown following colorectal surgery despite diligently following all skincare guidelines, including using a barrier layer at all times (Figure 18.23). Prescription triple paste (zinc oxide 40% (Desitin 30 g in tube), cholestyramine 4 g per scoop, and nystatin powder 10,000 units/g 15-gram container) is a very effective cream, but many other creams and ointments are available. When there is a concern for a yeast infection, nystatin ointment is the key first step. The nystatin ointment (anti-fungal) should be placed first to ensure the medicated cream is on the skin, followed by the barrier layers to prevent friction.

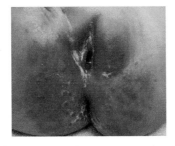

Figure 18.23 Perineum of a similar patient with a severe perineal rash.

Other good options are zinc oxide 40% (Desitin), clotrimazole (anti-fungal), and stoma powder, which are all over-the-counter treatments that can be mixed to create a similar paste without requiring a prescription and, therefore, present less of a financial burden (Figure 18.24).

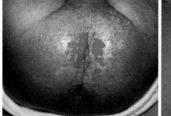 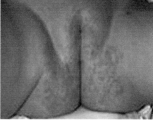

Figure 18.24 Perineal excoriation before and two weeks after the described care in a similar case.

After a PSARP, transanal pull-through, or stoma closure, perineal excoriation can be a real problem. Care of the perineum should start in the immediate postoperative period. Apply Cavilon Advanced™ or Marathon™ in the operating room at the end of the case or when the patient has returned to the surgical floor. This acts as a barrier to protect the skin. Preventative products should be placed at the bedside to cleanse and protect the skin. These products include a soft cleanser, dry wipes, and barrier creams. Provide the family with supplies for home to help treat and prevent diaper dermatitis and the algorithm of when to use the products (Figure 18.25).

SKIN CARE GUIDELINES FOR THE COLORECTAL PATIENT

Careful attention to skin care is very important for colorectal patients. After surgery the stool will be loose and the increased frequency of bowel movements can be irritating to the skin. Your child will require frequent diaper changes with good skin care.

SKIN BREAKDOWN PREVENTION PLAN:

1. Clean with warm water and mild soap.
2. Pat dry with dry cloth, do not wipe.
3. Apply Cavilon No-Sting Wipe on the skin.
4. Apply layer of Hydraguard or another skin barrier cream on top of the Cavilon.
5. Do NOT use baby wipes as they can cause irritation.

MILD SKIN BREAKDOWN TREATMENT PLAN:

1. Clean with warm water and mild soap.
2. Pat dry with dry cloth, do not wipe.
3. Apply Cavilon No-Sting Wipe on the skin.
4. Apply layer of Z-guard or Zinc based diaper cream on top of the Cavilon.
5. Do NOT use baby wipes as they can further irritate the skin, causing more breakdown.

MODERATE TO SEVERE SKIN BREAKDOWN TREATMENT PLAN: (If skin is open, bleeding, wet or weepy)

1. Cleanse with warm water and mild soap.
2. Pat dry with dry cloth, do not wipe.
   - **1st:** Apply a dusting of stoma-adhesive powder to clean skin.
   - **2nd:** Apply the Cavilon No-Sting Wipe to set the powder creating a crusting effect.
   - **3rd:** Apply layer of Triple Butt Paste (You will need a prescription).
   - **Finally,** you can place a layer of non-adherent dressings such as Vaseline gauze or telfa on each buttock to help hold the creams in place and keep the stool off the area.
3. Do NOT use baby wipes as they can further irritate the skin, causing more breakdown

IMPORTANT NOTES:

- If cleared by the colorectal team you may put your child in the tub with warm water and gentle soap. This will help clean the skin and remove all the products.

- Try to only wipe off the top layer of cream during diaper changes and reapply ointment as needed. Do not scrub to get old cream off of the buttocks!

Figure 18.25

Note: "Triple Butt Paste" consists of desitin, nystatin, and cholestyramine.

RECOMMENDED READING

Krois, Wilfried, et al. A technique to reconstruct the anal sphincters following iatrogenic stretching related to a pull-through for Hirschsprung disease. *J Pediatr Surg.* 2021; 56(6): 1242–1246.

CHAPTER 19

LAXATIVES

TIMING OF STIMULANT LAXATIVES FOR AN EFFECTIVE BOWEL MANAGEMENT PLAN

Laxatives and stool softeners can be an effective treatment for children with constipation and soiling who have the anatomic elements to achieve continence (Figure 19.1). Most stimulant laxative medications (those containing Senna or bisacodyl) provoke a bowel movement within 8–12 hours of taking them. This time can vary slightly from child to child, so it is necessary to trial the medication first to see its effect. Stool softeners soften the stool; they do not provoke a bowel movement.

> Every day is a school day.
>
> – Michael Caty

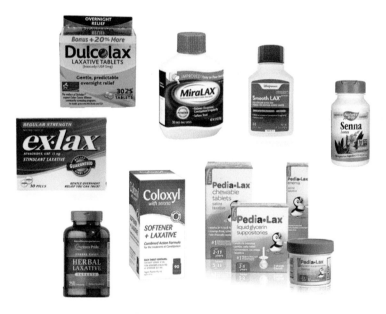

Figure 19.1 A variety of stool softeners and laxatives.

Once an estimated time to stool production is determined, the next step is to determine the best time of day for the child to have uninterrupted time on the toilet to have a bowel movement. For some, the medication is given in the morning to elicit a bowel movement once the child has finished school. Others may take it before bed to elicit a bowel movement in the morning upon waking. This is an important conversation to have with the child and their family, to work out a plan that suits the family best.

Usually stimulant laxatives alone with water soluble fiber create a good bowel movement pattern, 1–2 stools per day. Sometimes a softener is added to achieve the ideal stool consistency.

DOI: 10.1201/9781003150015-22

CHAPTER 20

THICKENING THE STOOL WITH FIBER

FIBER SUPPLEMENTATION

For patients switching from retrograde enemas or ante-grade flushes to laxatives, it is helpful to start them on water-soluble fiber at least 3 days before their first dose of laxatives (Figure 20.1). Laxatives will "push" stool through the colon, but will do so at a rate that prevents the body from absorbing enough water from the colon. The stool, therefore, becomes more liquid. By adding

> As a surgeon worrying about my patients, I'm always uncomfortable. I've just become comfortable being uncomfortable.
>
> **– Contributed by: Payam Saadai**

water-soluble fiber to the regimen, the stool will be less watery and have more bulk (Figure 20.2). The addition of fiber makes the stool more formed and consolidates the number of bowel movements. With better stool consistency and a decreased number of bowel movements, the patient has a better capacity for bowel control, because they can feel the formed stool in their rectum (proprioception).

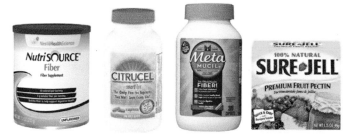

Figure 20.1 Fiber supplement options.

TYPE	DOSAGE AND USE	WHERE TO FIND IT
Pectin (Sure-Jell®)	1 Tablespoon = 2 grams of fiber	Found in the grocery store In the jelly/canning section or online at www.pacificpectin.com Get the sugar-free version.
Citrucel®	Powder 1 Tablespoon = 2 grams of fiber Capsule 2 capsules = 1 gram of fiber	Found in the pharmacy section of the store or online at www.citrucel.com You can use the generic or the brand name. Get the sugar-free version.
Metamucil® (psyllium husk)	Powder 1 Teaspoon = 2 grams of fiber Capsule 5 capsules = 2 grams of fiber Wafer 1 packet (2 wafers) = 3 grams of fiber	Found in the pharmacy section of the store or online at www.metamucil.com Get the sugar-free version.
Nutrisource® (guar gum)	1 Tablespoon (scoop) = 3 grams of fiber *Can be sprinkled on food or mixed in drinks.	Found in the pharmacy section of the store, online, or through homecare companies.

Figure 20.2 Fiber supplement dosing.

HELPING CHILDREN TAKE THEIR FIBER

Forget the mistake, remember the
lesson.

– Contributed by: Bu Nguyen

Water-soluble fiber is an important part of many patients' bowel regimens (Figure 20.3). It helps add bulk to the stool, allowing patients to have less frequent stools and better sensation. Unfortunately, fiber can be difficult for some children to take on a daily basis. Many fibers have a bad taste or change the consistency of what they are mixed in.

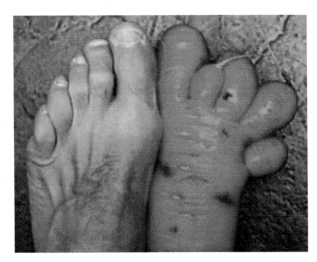

Figure 20.3 Funny photo of what happens when one takes too much fiber.

Here are some tips to make it easier for parents:

- Mix the fiber in the child's favorite drink or try mixing it in a thicker beverage such as a smoothie or milk shake. Always make sure the volume of liquid that the fiber is mixed in is a volume the child will finish.
- Try mixing the fiber in foods, such as applesauce, pudding, yogurt, or ice cream.
- It may be helpful if the child does not know the fiber has been mixed in.
- Try different brands, flavors, and forms of the supplement. Some fibers come in capsules or wafers. Fiber gummies are *not* recommended as there is little to no bulking effect.
- Do not let the fiber sit out for a long time before the child finishes it. It will cause the drink to thicken.

CHAPTER 21

BACTERIAL OVERGROWTH

SMALL INTESTINAL BACTERIAL OVERGROWTH

Small intestinal bacterial overgrowth (SIBO) is an imbalance in the microbiome of the small intestine. Various mechanisms can cause SIBO, but it is generally related to decreased motility and/or obstructions and is commonly seen in HD patients. This microbiome imbalance can lead to a reduction in normal flora and an increase in potentially pathogenic bacteria.

When there is no indication – there is complication.

– Contributed by: Inbal Samuk

Clinical manifestations of SIBO include weight loss, dehydration, diarrhea, and nutritional deficiencies. Patients with HD and SIBO may have a presentation similar to that of enterocolitis, with abdominal pain and distension requiring irrigations to empty. These episodes may be recurrent and may come back after completion of a course of antibiotics.

SIBO is best treated by an alternating antibiotic regimen, such as metronidazole and/or amoxicillin.

Symptoms of SIBO	
Gastrointestinal symptoms	General symptoms
Abdominal pain	Malnutrition
Diarrhea	Weight loss
Bloating	Growth stunting
Flatulence	Megaloblastic, macrocytic anemia (vitamin B_{12} deficiency)
Steatorrhea	Fat-soluble vitamin deficiency (A, D, and E)
Carbohydrate malabsorption	Hypoproteinemia
	Increased risk of bloodstream infection in children with SBS

Abbreviations: SBS = short bowel syndrome; SIBO = small intestinal bacterial overgrowth

Figure 21.1

RECOMMENDED READING

Sieczkowska A, Ladowski P, Kaminska B, Lifschitz C. Small bowel bacterial overgrowth in children. *J Pediatr Gastroenterol Nutr.* 2016; 62(2): 197–207.

Chapter 22

SHARING TISSUES

SPLIT APPENDIX TECHNIQUE

Depending on the length of the appendix, it can be used for both a Malone and a Mitrofanoff. The split appendix technique can be used to divide the appendix. A minimum of 5–7 cm is required to create a Mitrofanoff. A minimum of 2 cm is required to create a Malone. If the abdominal wall is very thick, additional length may be required. Depending on the total length of the appendix, the appendix can be divided according to Figure 22.1.

> Keep your eye on the donut, not the hole.
>
> **– Michael Caty**

The panel of pictures in Figure 22.2 shows a 7 cm appendix being split, using the split appendix technique, with the distal 5 cm allocated to the creation of a Mitrofanoff and the proximal 2 cm used to create the Malone. The plication of the Malone is shown in the final panel.

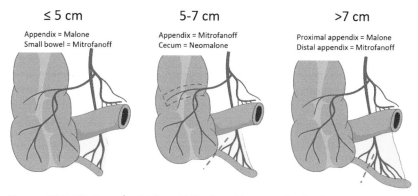

Figure 22.1 Options for Malone/Mitrofanoff appendix sharing.

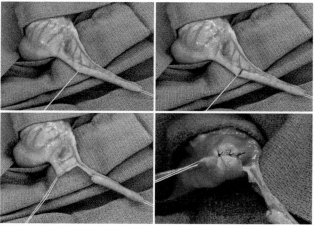

Figure 22.2 Split appendix technique.

DOI: 10.1201/9781003150015-25

RECOMMENDED READING

Halleran DR, Sloots CEJ, Fuller MK, Diefenbach K. Adjuncts to bowel management for fecal incontinence and constipation, the role of surgery: Appendicostomy, cecostomy, neoappendicostomy, and colonic resection. *Semin Pediatr Surg.* 2020 Dec; 29(6): 150998.

VanderBrink BA, Levitt MA, Defoor WR, Alam S. Creation of an appendicovesicostomy Mitrofanoff from a preexisting appendicocecostomy utilizing the spilt appendix technique. *J Pediatr Surg.* 2014 Apr; 49(4): 656–659.

USING THE SIGMOID COLON FOR BLADDER AUGMENTATION

For a patient who needs a urologic reconstruction, one should always know the bowel status first to create a collaborative surgical reconstructive plan that addresses both the urinary and bowel management needs of the patient. An example of such a patient would be a patient with spina bifida who needs a bladder augmentation. In evaluating bowel and bladder management needs, attempt to answer the following questions:

- Is the colon easy or challenging to empty?
- What regimen is needed?
- How much time does it take to empty the colon?

If the sigmoid colon is redundant or dilated and the patient is requiring a high laxative dose, a concentrated flush, or extended time to evacuate the colon, the sigmoid colon can be used to augment the bladder (Figure 22.3). The sigmoid colon is removed from the fecal stream, but its mesentery is kept intact. The segment of the sigmoid is then rolled over to augment the bladder. The sigmoid colon above and below the graft is then anastomosed. The effective "sigmoid resection" then improves the efficacy of the antegrade flush, reducing the potency and sit time required for antegrade flushes.

> When you reach the end of your rope, tie a knot in it and hang on.
>
> **– Franklin D. Roosevelt, Contributed by: Teresa Russell**

> No matter how far down the wrong road you have gone you can still turn back.
>
> **– Fred Ryckman**

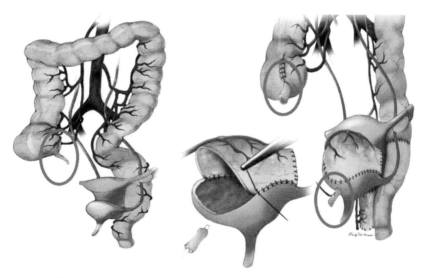

Figure 22.3 Bladder augmentation using the sigmoid colon.

CHAPTER 23

FUNCTIONAL CONSTIPATION AND FECAL INCONTINENCE MYTHS

MYTH: A CHILD LOSES THE ABILITY TO DEVELOP BOWEL CONTROL ONCE ENEMAS ARE INITIATED

Parents have a certain degree of reluctance to accept a bowel routine, especially rectal enemas, as a treatment for fecal incontinence, based on several misconceptions. Among these is the mistaken belief that a child loses bowel control or that the child becomes dependent on rectal therapy for life. If the patient was born with a type

> If you want to steer the ship, you have to stay at the helm.
>
> **– Contributed by: Marc Levitt**

of malformation that has a poor prognosis, then a child may indeed require enemas/flushes for life. However, a patient born with an ARM who has good potential for bowel control can use enemas for bowel management temporarily. After 6 months to 1 year, treatment may be converted to oral laxatives, and the patient can be allowed to realize their potential for bowel control and demonstrate their capacity for voluntary bowel movements.

Some parents may believe that subjecting their child to bowel management with enemas may interfere with the natural toilet training process, which is also incorrect. Proper bowel management may actually help the patient become toilet trained, because the child can sense stool in the now-empty rectum, improve their urinary control, and learn the desirable feeling of being fresh and clean.

RECOMMENDED READING

Nash O, Choueiki JM, Levitt MA, eds. *Fecal Incontinence and Constipation in Children: Case Studies.* 1st ed. CRC Press; 2019.

MYTH: CHILDREN WITH SEVERE CONSTIPATION AND FAILURE OF MEDICAL MANAGEMENT NEED A SIGMOID RESECTION

Only the sled dog in the first row gets the fresh breeze of the day. (translated from German)

– Contributed by: Martin Lacher

Colonic resection for functional constipation should not be considered a first-line intervention. Because of the collaboration between surgeons and GI/motility experts, we can now be more thoughtful about the decision to resect the colon. It is essential to treat the patient rather than imaging. The vast majority of patients who have failed medical management respond to a trial of antegrade flushes. If they do not respond, only then should they be considered for a colonic resection. The decision should be based on a motility evaluation to help objectively demonstrate which part of the colon should be removed. Motility studies include a sitzmark study, nuclear scintigraphy, and colonic manometry (CMAN). Indications for resection include poor response to medical management with antegrade flushes and a discrete colonic segment with dysmotility or a significantly dilated or redundant rectosigmoid colon that interferes with the effectiveness of antegrade flushes. Resection can also be considered in older children and young adults with chronic constipation who have done well with antegrade flushes but fail to transition to oral laxatives and no longer wish to depend on antegrade flushes. In cases in which severe constipation leads to failure to thrive (FTT), an ileostomy should be considered. Of course, in all cases anal sphincter and pelvic floor dysfunction must first be checked for and treated. Surgical management options for patients who have failed medical management are detailed in Figure 23.1.

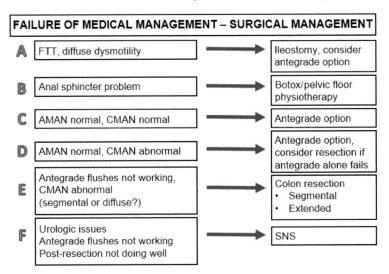

Figure 23.1 Surgical alternatives, focusing on recently published data. AMAN: anorectal manometry; CMAN: colonic manometry; FTT: failure to thrive; SNS: sacral nerve stimulation.

RECOMMENDED READING

Gasior A, Reck C, Vilanova-Sanchez A, Diefenbach KA, Yacob D, Lu P, Vaz K, Di Lorenzo C, Levitt MA, Wood RJ. Surgical management of functional constipation: An intermediate report of a new approach using a laparoscopic sigmoid resection combined with Malone appendicostomy. *J Pediatr Surg.* 2018 Jun; 53(6): 1160–1162.

Wood RJ, Yacob D, Levitt MA. Surgical options for the management of severe functional constipation in children. *Curr Opin Pediatr.* 2016 Jun; 28(3): 370–379.

MYTH: PATIENTS MUST BE SUCCESSFUL WITH RECTAL ENEMAS BEFORE GETTING A MALONE

Indications for a Malone antegrade continence enema (MACE) include difficulties with stooling and bowel control in patients with ARM, HD, spinal diagnoses, and functional constipation with overflow incontinence. There is contention in the literature around the idea that a MACE procedure should be offered to such patients only

> The word 'happiness' would lose its meaning if it were not balanced by sadness.
>
> **– Carl Gustav Jung**

after they have successfully achieved social continence through a regimen of enemas given rectally. In these reports, success is defined as absolute cleanliness with no accidents between enemas.

However, there are several situations in which a child may be unable to tolerate rectal therapy, and, therefore, a Malone appendicostomy is a reasonable first step. Examples include a child with a low continence potential ARM who is anally defensive or a patient who seeks independence and cannot physically self-administer a rectal enema. In such cases, an antegrade option can be provided with a bowel management regimen developed thereafter. Of course, it is the flush cocktail itself, not the route of administration, that is the key to a successful BMP.

RECOMMENDED READING

Halleran DR, Sloots CEJ, Fuller MK, Diefenbach K. Adjuncts to bowel management for fecal incontinence and constipation, the role of surgery: Appendicostomy, cecostomy, neoappendicostomy, and colonic resection. *Semin Pediatr Surg.* 2020 Dec; 29(6): 150998.

Halleran DR, Vilanova-Sanchez A, Rentea RM, Vriesman MH, Maloof T, Lu PL, Onwuka A, Weaver L, Vaz KK, Yacob D, Di Lorenzo C, Levitt MA, Wood RJ. A comparison of Malone appendicostomy and cecostomy for antegrade access as adjuncts to a bowel management program for patients with functional constipation or fecal incontinence. *J Pediatr Surg.* 2019 Jan; 54(1): 123–128.

Rangel SJ, Lawal TA, Bischoff A, Chatoorgoon K, Louden E, Peña A, Levitt MA. The appendix as a conduit for antegrade continence enemas in patients with anorectal malformations: Lessons learned from 163 cases treated over 18 years. *J Pediatr Surg.* 2011 Jun; 46(6): 1236–1242.

MYTH: SENNA IS PROBLEMATIC BECAUSE PATIENTS DEVELOP TOLERANCE TO IT

You can learn new things at any time in your life if you're willing to be a beginner. If you actually learn to like being a beginner, the whole world opens up to you.

– Barbara Sher

The primary mechanism of senna is selective action at the nerve plexus of intestinal smooth muscle, increasing intestinal motility. Many clinicians avoid senna for reasons such as tolerance or side effects, but these concerns have been found to have little scientific justification. A literature review of pediatric senna side effects demonstrated no tolerance in children with long-term utilization.

Abdominal cramps, vomiting, and diarrhea were found in a third of patients. Of the patients studied, 53% required adjustments in the dose of senna, 37% of which (241 patients) increased the dose in the last 3 years, and 17.1% (110/640) needed a decrease in the dose. The increase in dosage was thought to be due to normal child growth and unrelated to tolerance. No patient increased the dose and needed to stop the treatment owing to tolerance. Additionally, senna-induced dermatitis is a rare side effect, seen in 2.2% of patients, and is correlated with higher doses of senna and prolonged skin contact with stool (Figure 23.2). Melanosis coli has been seen in adults on chronic senna. It is a darkening of the mucosa with no clinical implication.

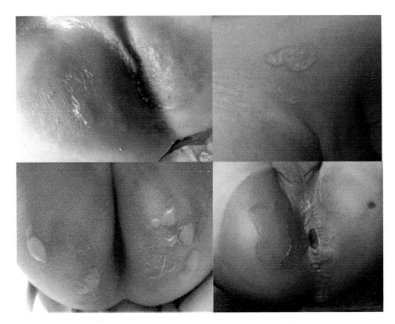

Figure 23.2 Senna rash variations.

RECOMMENDED READING

Vilanova-Sanchez A, Gasior AC, Toocheck N, Weaver L, Wood RJ, Reck CA, Wagner A, Hoover E, Gagnon R, Jaggers J, Maloof T, Nash O, Williams C, Levitt MA. Are senna-based laxatives safe when used as long-term treatment for constipation in children? *J Pediatr Surg.* 2018 Apr; 53(4): 722–727.

MYTH: X-RAYS ARE NOT HELPFUL IN BOWEL MANAGEMENT PATIENTS AND THE RADIATION IS DANGEROUS

An abdominal X-ray is very helpful to assess residual stool burden and track the efficacy of therapy (Figure 23.3). The goal of treatment is for patients to empty their colon daily and be free of soiling. Treatment regimens are adjusted based on the child's clinical and radiographic responses. For a patient with soiling two to three times per day, the soiling could be due to an inadequate enema, which failed to clean the colon, or the accidents could be due to overstimulation by an enema that is too strong. Only an X-ray can make the determination as to which of the scenarios is occurring. The treatment plan is considered successful when the abdominal radiograph is clear of stool in the rectum, sigmoid, and left colon, and the child has no soiling. In a study of pediatric gastroenterologists, nearly one-half changed their management based on the imaging findings.

> The only thing worse than a blind believer is a seeing denier.
>
> **– Alberto Peña**

Parents often raise concerns about radiation exposure. The radiation dose of single abdominal X-ray is about 0.7 mSv. Higher radiation exposure occurs in the course of daily life or while in an airplane. On average, the radiation dose from natural background sources is about 3.0 mSv per year. The selective use of X-rays to assess the adequacy of a child's bowel regimen is highly effective and poses little risk to the patient.

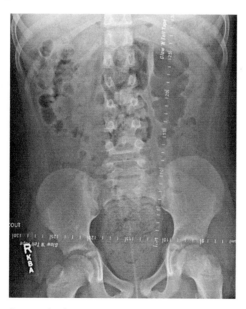

Figure 23.3 Abdominal radiograph demonstrating a large rectosigmoid stool burden.

RECOMMENDED READING

Beinvogl B, Sabharwal S, McSweeney M, Nurko S. Are we using abdominal radiographs appropriately in the management of pediatric constipation? *J Pediatr.* 2017 Dec; 191: 179–183.

EPA (United States Environmental Protection Agency), Radiation Protection, "How much radiation am I exposed to when I get a medical x-ray procedure?". www.epa.gov/radiation/how-much-radiation-am-i-exposed-when-i-get-medical-x-ray-procedure

PART IV

POST-PSARP AND POST-HD PULL-THROUGH PROBLEMS

CHAPTER 24

PROBLEMS AFTER PSARP

EVALUATION OF THE PATIENT WITH AN ANORECTAL MALFORMATION WHO WAS PREVIOUSLY REPAIRED BUT IS NOT DOING WELL

After an ARM repair in a patient who is not doing well, the first step is to assess the patient's potential for continence. The clinician evaluating such a patient can then collect more anatomic information with a full imaging workup, including a pelvic MRI, to evaluate for a remnant of the original fistula (ROOF) and the trajectory of the pull-through, and a contrast enema, to evaluate for any stricture or dilation in the pulled through colon. Then, the patient should proceed to an EUA, often with an accompanying cystoscopy and/or vaginoscopy, to have their anatomy evaluated for any abnormalities that

> Your goal as a surgeon is to be a better internist than the internists - the corollary for pediatric surgeons would be - Your goal as a pediatric surgeon is to be a better pediatrician than the pediatricians.
>
> **– Bernie Langer, hepatobiliary surgeon and father of Jack Langer**

would require a reoperation, such as an anal mislocation, stricture, ROOF, or rectal prolapse. If abnormal anatomy is found, then the surgeon should restore as normal anatomy as possible to the patient to maximize their potential for bowel control. They should also consider whether the patient could benefit from a Malone at the time of the reoperation to provide antegrade access and mechanical cleaning of the colon while the patient develops bowel control using their restored anatomy. If the anatomy is good and no surgical intervention is required, then the patient can proceed with a bowel management program (BMP) that would either involve a laxative trial or an enema regimen (Figure 24.1).

DOI: 10.1201/9781003150015-28

> Tie the knot to the baby, not the baby to the knot.
>
> **– Contributed by: Michael Phillips**

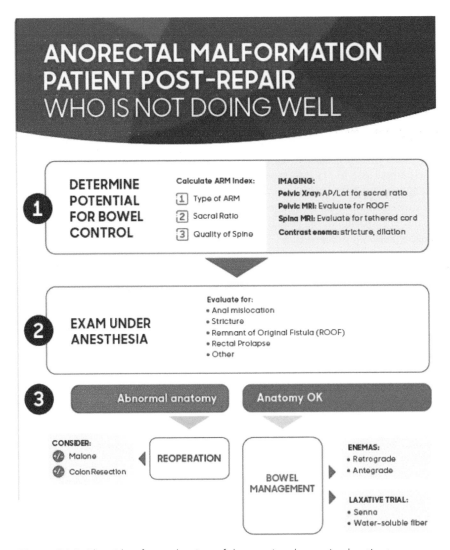

Figure 24.1 Algorithm for evaluation of the previously repaired patient.

RECOMMENDED READING

Lane VA, Calisto J, de Blaauw I, Calkins CM, Samuk I, Avansino JR. Assessing the previously repaired patient with an anorectal malformation who is not doing well. *Semin Pediatr Surg.* 2020 Dec; 29(6): 150995.

SIGMOID RESECTION IN AN ANORECTAL MALFORMATION PATIENT

It is very rare that an ARM patient would require a sigmoid resection. A sigmoid resection may be needed in a patient with mega rectosigmoid and severe constipation that is not manageable by laxatives, enemas, or antegrade flushes (Figure 24.2). In such a case, saving the rectal reservoir is vital for continence. So, to remove the

> I have not failed. I've just found 10,000 ways that won't work.
>
> **– Thomas Edison**

sigmoid, do not ligate the sigmoid arcade. Remember, the distal rectum may have been dissected at the original ARM pull-through. Therefore, the inferior and middle hemorrhoidal blood supply likely does not exist, and the rectum is perfused by the superior hemorrhoidal artery which originates from the inferior mesenteric artery (IMA). The IMA arcade may have been compromised at the time of the colostomy creation. Thus, if such a patient needs a sigmoid resection, make sure to transect the upper rectum/lower sigmoid high enough (just above the peritoneal reflection) so that mesenteric blood supply can be visualized going deep into the pelvis for the supply of blood to the rectum (Figures 24.3 and 24.4).

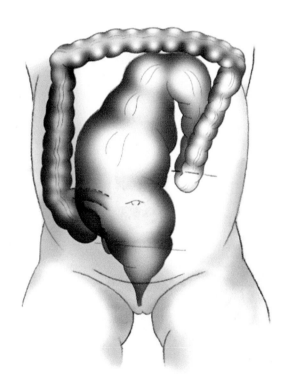

Figure 24.2

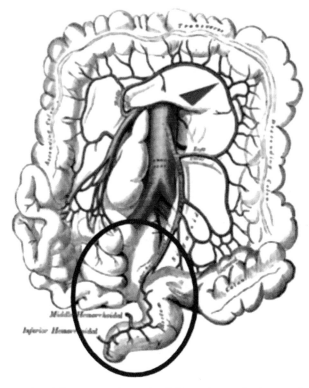

Figure 24.3 Blood supply of the rectum from the IMA and superior hemorrhoidal artery.

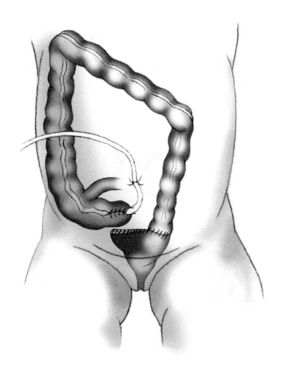

Figure 24.4 Sigmoid resection, preservation of the rectum, Malone appendicostomy.

MANAGING A SKIN LEVEL ANAL STRICTURE

An HM anoplasty, shown in Figure 24.5, is a great solution for a skin-level stricture. Sutures are placed at the 2, 4, 8, and 10 o'clock positions around the anal opening on mosquito clamps. As the sutures are held up, a radial incision is placed between them. The radial incision then creates a longitudinal orientation when the mosquito clamps are pulled apart. The mucosa of the bowel is sutured to the skin longitudinally, utilizing an interrupted long-term absorbable suture. A narrow anal opening, such as a Hegar size 8, can be converted to a size 16 utilizing the HM anoplasty. The technique only works for a short (2–3 mm) area of narrowing. This technique can also be used for a congenital anal stenosis at the skin level.

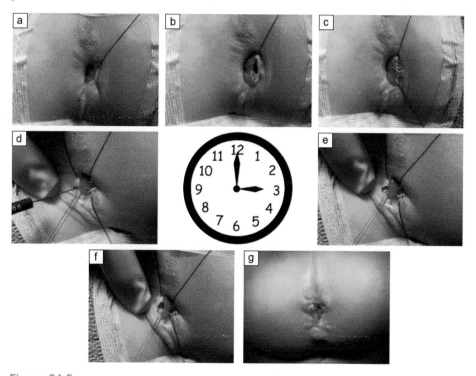

Figure 24.5

The steps of an HM anoplasty are shown in Figure 24.5, as outlined below:

(a) Sutures at 2 and 4 o'clock.
(b) Radial incision cut and stretched to set up longitudinal suture line.
(c) Longitudinal sutures placed.
(d) Radial cut between 8 and 10 o'clock.
(e) Cut between 8 and 10 o'clock.
(f) Stretched skin, showing longitudinal repair.
(g) Completed HM anoplasty.

RECOMMENDED READING

Halleran DR, Sanchez AV, Rentea RM, et al. Assessment of the Heineke-Mikulicz anoplasty for skin level postoperative anal strictures and congenital anal stenosis. *J Pediatr Surg.* 2019 Jan; 54(1): 118–122.

RECTAL BLEEDING: IS THE RECTAL PROLAPSE THE SOURCE?

The presence of a rectal prolapse in a patient with an ARM after surgical repair should not be automatically blamed as the cause of rectal bleeding.

A 13-month-old female with a history of an ARM with rectovestibular fistula and distal vaginal atresia who had previously undergone a PSARP presented 10 months postoperatively with bleeding per rectum and new-onset bloody stools. At baseline she was known to have a small rectal prolapse with blood-streaked diapers (approximately two per month). The mother noted that over the past couple of days, there was an increase in bright red blood per rectum in the diaper. She brought the patient in for evaluation after she had an acute, large episode of black, tarry stool, and surgery was consulted owing to the patient's surgical history.

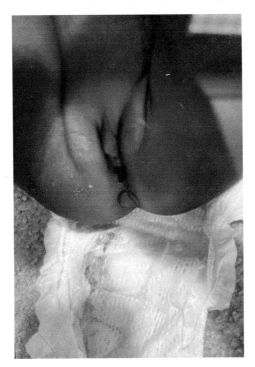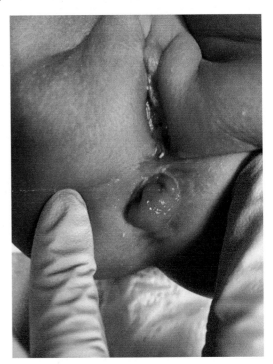

Figure 24.6 Rectal prolapse with diaper streaked with blood.

The patient otherwise appeared well, had been tolerating feeds, continued to have an appropriate number of wet diapers, and was behaving normally. On evaluation, the patient had normal vital signs with a soft, nondistended abdomen, along with a healthy, pink rectal prolapse without concerning findings or recent stigmata of bleeding (Figure 24.6). Lab work was significant for a drop in hemoglobin over time from the last recorded hemoglobin of 17.6 to 12.2, with a normal MCV. The recommendation was to obtain GI consultation, a Meckel's scan, EGD, and to perform a colonoscopy. Streaking of the diaper or underwear can occur with this type of prolapse, and this may need to be surgically trimmed, but, in this case, the more significant bleeding is almost definitely due to a different cause. In this case that cause was gastritis noted on EGD.

MYTH: ANORECTAL MALFORMATION PATIENTS WITH A LOST RECTUM WHO UNDERWENT A PULL-THROUGH OF THEIR COLOSTOMY CANNOT BE CONTINENT

Bowel control requires sensation, sphincter control, rectosigmoid motility, and reservoir function. For children with ARM, rectal loss may result from a rectum that was discarded at the time of PSARP. This is a situation that should be avoided but that may occur if the blood supply to a high distal rectum is lost. This could occur if the original colostomy was placed too distal on the sigmoid and the surgeon could not save the rectal blood supply. On contrast enema imaging after the initial rectal operation, the clue to this anatomy is seeing colonic contractions down to the perineum with haustral markings (Figure 24.7). This means the patient has no rectum. Older operations before the PSARP, such as an abdominoperineal pull-through, did this rectal resection routinely.

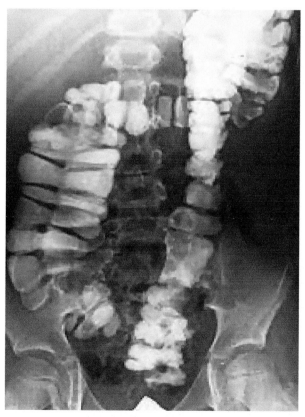

Figure 24.7 Contrast enema showing haustral markings in the neorectum which means the sigmoid was pulled through.

While the rectum acts as a reservoir, children without a rectum may still achieve continence as their potential is based on their original malformation, the quality of the spine, and the sacral ratio.

Those with good sphincters and a normal spine can achieve bowel control even without their rectum. They do need to feel the stretch of the neorectum, which clues them in to the need to contract their external sphincters.

FREE AIR AFTER COLOSTOMY CLOSURE

A baby boy, born with an ARM, underwent initial colostomy and subsequent PSARP. At the age of 7 months, he underwent his colostomy closure. The anus was a good size, without stricture or prolapse. He did well at first, starting to stool on day 2 and was able to eat and be discharged home. On postoperative day 5, he returned to the emergency room (ER) with fever, abdominal distension, and tenderness. An abdominal X-ray performed in the ER is shown in Figure 24.8.

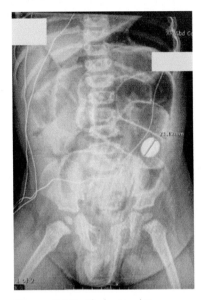

Figure 24.8 Abdominal X-ray.

What do you think is going on? What would you do?

The X-ray shows a bowel obstruction and free air, with a foreign body in the left lower quadrant. The foreign body turned out to be a swallowed battery, sitting at the anastomosis, which had caused a perforation (Figure 24.9). A laparotomy, washout, and new colostomy were needed.

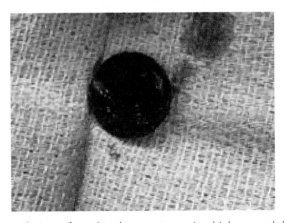

Figure 24.9 Disc battery that was found at the anastomosis which caused the perforation.

MYTH: A REDO PSARP IS ONLY FOR PATIENTS WITH GOOD POTENTIAL FOR BOWEL CONTROL

It is a myth that a child with an ARM, a poor sacrum, and a poor spine should not be offered a redo to correct an anal mislocation or any other problem, because it will not change their potential for bowel control.

> The most important year of my training was my first year in practice.
>
> **– Dave Wesson**

Patients with a previously repaired ARM can suffer from complications that lead to incontinence. In a study of 153 reoperative PSARPs, mislocation (61%) and stricture (36%) were the most common indications. Reoperation can improve anatomic and functional outcomes, even in those with poor potential for continence. Interestingly, in the same study of 153 children post-redo, 79/153 (52%) had a poor potential for bowel control (Figure 24.10). Of those 79 with poor potential, 24 (30%) were on laxatives only and 55 (70%) were on enemas. 16/24 (67%) taking laxatives were continent of stool and 42/55 (76%) using enemas were clean. Additionally, most (80%) of those with good potential for bowel control developed voluntary bowel movements. Quality of Life and Baylor Continence scores improved in the vast majority of patients.

Therefore, a redo should be offered if the original PSARP can be anatomically improved for reasons such as anal mislocation, rectal stricture, rectal prolapse, or ROOF.

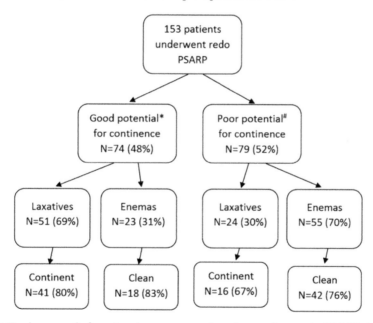

Figure 24.10 Twelve-month functional outcomes of patients after redo PSARP. * Patients with good potential for continence include patients with a normally developed sacrum (SR ≥ 0.70) and no spinal anomaly. # Patients considered to have poor potential for continence include those with sacral hypo-development (SR < 0.70), an associated spinal anomaly (e.g. tethered cord, fatty filum, or myelomeningocele), or both (from Wood RJ et al., 2020).

RECOMMENDED READING

Wood RJ, Halleran DR, Ahmad H, et al. Assessing the benefit of reoperations in patients who suffer from fecal incontinence after repair of their anorectal malformation. *J Pediatr Surg.* 2020 Oct; 55(10): 2159–2165.

CHAPTER 25

DECIDING WHEN TO DO A REDO PROCEDURE IN ARM

POSTERIOR MISLOCATION AND GOOD POTENTIAL FOR BOWEL CONTROL

A 5-year-old female with a prior ARM repair for rectovestibular fistula presents to the clinic with daily soiling. She has a normal sacrum (lateral sacral ratio 0.9) and a normal spine. Her exam is shown in Figure 25.1.

Le mieux est l'ennemi du bien. The perfect is the enemy of good.

– Voltaire

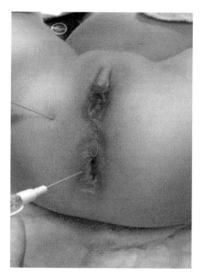

Figure 25.1 Posterior mislocation of the anoplasty, original malformation was a rectovestibular fistula. The blue dot marks the correct location for the anoplasty.

Would you do a redo PSARP or not? If so, what is the indication for the redo?

With a rectovestibular fistula, a good sacrum, and a lateral sacral ratio of 0.9, this child has an excellent potential for bowel control.

From the photo, it is clear that the anus is posteriorly mislocated. The surrounding scarring may suggest a wound dehiscence at the initial PSARP. The pink ellipse anterior to the current location of the anus is the correct center of the sphincters. In this case, this was confirmed by an electrical stimulation test. Therefore, a redo PSARP is needed.

If you decided to do surgery, how would you manage the patient postoperatively?

Don't play poker with someone else's chips.

— **Michael Caty**

A redo would entail moving the anoplasty anteriorly and closing the location where the anus is currently located. A colostomy is not needed in such cases. However, keeping the patient on clear liquids only for 5 days postoperatively allows for good perineal healing by reducing pressure of formed stool on the healing perineal incision. Once good perineal healing is ensured, the diet can be advanced. Depending on the age of the patient, placing a Malone at the same time as the redo would give the child a chance to get mechanically clean and to facilitate the achievement of bowel control as they learn how to control their improved anal anatomy.

POSTERIOR MISLOCATION AND GOOD POTENTIAL FOR BOWEL CONTROL

A 12-year-old boy presents to the clinic with soiling. The patient was born with an ARM and had a colostomy and PSARP done during the first year of life followed by colostomy closure. He also had a tethered cord, which has been detethered. The lateral sacral ratio is 0.33. In the photos in Figure 25.2 you see the current anatomy, and, in the second panel, the white dot is where the center of the sphincter maps with electrical stimulation.

How would you manage this patient with a posterior mislocation and rectal prolapse?

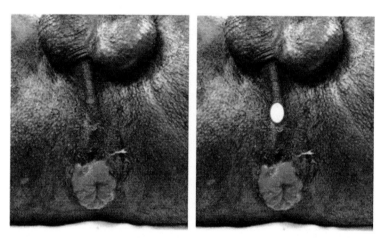

Figure 25.2 Posterior anal mislocation and rectal prolapse.

This child requires a full workup for a postoperative ARM patient who is not doing well. This should include renal and bladder ultrasounds, a spinal MRI, a pelvic MRI, a VCUG, an EUA, a cystoscopy, and consideration for urodynamics (UDS) testing based on the patient's urinary status, given his history of tethered spinal cord. Both pelvic MRI and cystoscopy are crucial to rule out a ROOF.

From the photo and electrical stimulation test results, it is obvious that the anus is prolapsed and posteriorly mislocated. He needs a redo for practical reasons – the prolapse is likely causing trouble for him with bleeding and mucus production – and, at the same time, the anoplasty can be moved to the center of the sphincters. Although the patient has a poor potential for continence, the redo offers a small chance for him to achieve voluntary bowel movements, and will at least solve the prolapse. Placing a Malone appendicostomy at the same time for antegrade flushes would be an ideal adjunct.

REMNANT OF THE ORIGINAL RECTAL FISTULA

A 6-year-old male had an ARM which was previously repaired. After his colostomy closure, the patient suffered from multiple urinary tract infections (UTIs) and renal damage from presumed neurogenic bladder. He ultimately underwent a kidney transplant. He had also undergone two repairs for rectal prolapse. This patient presents to the clinic after your evaluation for a previously repaired ARM patient with the MRI shown in Figure 25.3.

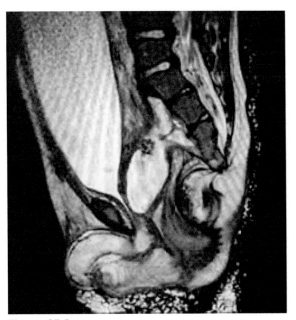

Figure 25.3

What is your diagnosis?

This is a ROOF, formerly called a posterior urethral diverticulum (PUD). The white structure behind the bladder neck is the old rectum that the surgeon never dissected. It can result from a transabdominal (laparoscopic) dissection of a lower fistula (rectoprostatic or rectobulbar). In this case, it seems to be entering at the lower prostatic level of the urethra. This could be a source of the UTIs, with contamination of the urinary tract by the bacteria present in the mucous of the rectal mucosa. Usually, these ROOFs lie between the pulled-through rectum and the urinary tract. Interestingly, here the ROOF is in that location, but rises alongside the rectum and is attached to the sacrum. The rectum must have been cut off at the original repair but left open, and that segment adhered to the sacrum. This ROOF can be removed through a posterior sagittal incision with the repair of the posterior urethra during the same operation. The procedure can be done laparoscopically as well, although the adherence to the sacrum would be challenging to dissect. After the anticipated improvement of the urinary function from removal of this infectious source, the patient will need urodynamics to assess his bladder function, followed by Malone and Mitrofanoff placement, if needed.

RECOMMENDED READING

Rentea RM, Halleran DR, Vilanova-Sanchez A, et al. Diagnosis and management of a remnant of the original fistula (ROOF) in males following surgery for anorectal malformations. *J Pediatr Surg.* 2019 Oct; 54(10): 1988–1992.

ANAL STRICTURE

A 6-year-old child with a history of ARM with rectovestibular fistula repaired in infancy has an anal stricture and severe constipation. She has had several impactions and soils daily from overflow owing to this constipation and stricture. The anoplasty is well located, and she has a good sacrum and a good spine status. The contrast study is shown in Figure 25.4.

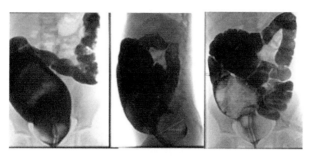

Figure 25.4 Contrast enema.

What would you do?

(a) Redo PSARP only to manage the stricture.
(b) Redo PSARP with additional removal of the distal dilated rectosigmoid followed by anastomosis of more normal caliber sigmoid to the neoanus.
(c) Redo PSARP to manage the stricture with a simultaneous Malone or cecostomy.

In this case, the patient has a well-located anus, a severe stricture, and a massively dilated rectosigmoid, with more a normal caliber proximal sigmoid. The key next step is to manage the stricture and create a Malone. With a better-sized anus and regular flushes, the colon will likely decompress, and no sigmoid resection will be needed.

Would your treatment plan be different if this were a 2-year-old or a 9-year-old?

The approach would be basically the same in both 2- and 9-year-old patients – fix the anus – but, in the older child, adding a Malone gets them clean quickly and helps rehabilitate the colon. The child will most likely not need the Malone in the long run because they should be able to develop bowel control.

If you just managed the stricture and did a Malone, and 6 months later you still cannot successfully empty the colon, what would you do?

If you would, at this point, remove some colon, which option would you choose?

(a) Rectosigmoid resection (like for an HD case).
(b) Sigmoid resection only, preserving the rectum.

Are there any specific considerations for such an operation?

If, 6 months after managing the stricture and creating a Malone, the dilated colon is still not successfully emptying, it now requires intervention. This situation would be extremely rare. Since the ARM patient without an anal canal is dependent on the rectal reservoir (and rectal stretch, i.e. proprioception) for bowel control, removing the rectum should be avoided. If the colon cannot empty despite laxatives, enemas, or antegrade flushes, only then should a sigmoid resection be performed. Usually this does the trick, and the rectum, although dilated, can be preserved and can empty. An alternative approach would be to do rectal tapering via a posterior sagittal incision As noted previously, if such a sigmoid resection is performed, the IMA branches to the neorectum must be carefully preserved.

LATERAL MISLOCATION AND REMNANT OF ORIGINAL FISTULA

If you give him a penny for his
thoughts, you'll get change.

– Contributed by: Marc Levitt

A 5-year-old boy with ARM presents with soiling. Findings from evaluations, including an EUA and a pelvic MRI, are shown in Figure 25.5.

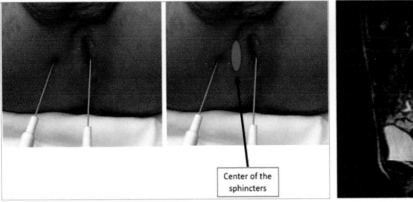

Center of the
sphincters

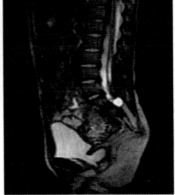

Figure 25.5 Exam showing a lateral mislocation of the anoplasty and an MRI showing a ROOF.

What is your assessment of this situation? What was the original malformation?

Evaluation of such patients should always include an EUA, cystoscopy, and imaging looking for any indications for reoperation. This patient has a lateral mislocation and a rectoprostatic ROOF. For the ARM patient who is not doing well, comprehensive evaluation is required to identify all potential complications before proceeding with revision surgery. Common indications for revision surgery include anal mislocation, stricture, prolapse, and ROOF.

In this case, a redo PSARP should be done to mobilize the rectum, remove the ROOF, repair the posterior urethra, and place the distal rectum in the center of the sphincters, passing it through the sphincters to correct the lateral mislocation.

RECOMMENDED READING

Ahmad H, Halleran DR, Maloof E, et al. Redo posterior sagittal anorectoplasty for lateral mislocation in patients with anorectal malformations. *J Pediatr Surg.* 2020 Nov; 55(11): 2521–2526.

POST-PSARP RECTAL PROLAPSE

A 10-month-old boy with ARM post-PSARP presents to the clinic with rectal prolapse. His exam is shown in Figure 25.6.

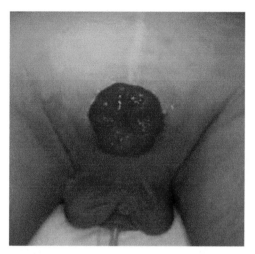

Figure 25.6 Rectal prolapse.

How would you manage this post-PSARP rectal prolapse? What technique would you use?
Can this case be done as an ambulatory procedure or does it require admission? Does this patient need a preoperative bowel preparation?

Note the circumferential nature of the prolapse and the flatness of the bottom. The child needs surgery because this prolapse affects his daily life by causing mucus discharge and recurrent bleeding from friction on his underwear. Prolapse can also interfere with the child's ability to close the anus, inhibiting his achievement of bowel control.

Assuming an EUA with electrical stimulation confirms that the anoplasty is in the correct location, a semicircumferential resection, followed by the resection of the other half a couple months later, works well. This will help to avoid a stricture and allow for ambulatory surgery in each case. The child can also avoid anal dilatations in the postoperative period. Some surgeons may prefer to admit for one night if they perform a full circumferential repair, which is also reasonable. But, given that this repair is at the skin level, a bowel preparation and a postoperative period of nil per os (NPO) are not necessary.

For this technique, start by placing stay sutures around the prolapsed tissue, excising the mucosa that is redundant, and then attaching the bowel with interrupted Vicryl sutures in a similar fashion to performing an anoplasty (Figure 25.7). Sometimes, for particularly bad prolapses, you need to do a redo PSARP with tacking of the posterior rectal wall to the muscle complex.

There's nothing more permanent than
a temporary solution to anything.

**– Siggie Ein, Contributed by: Jack
Langer**

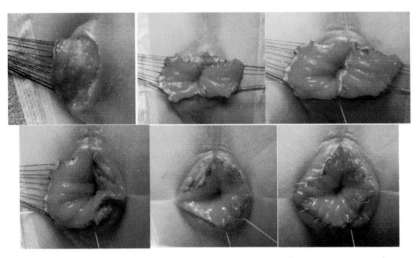

Figure 25.7 Technique for rectal prolapse repair, in this case a circumferential resection was performed.

POST-PSARP STRICTURE

Post-PSARP or post-redo PSARP constipation can be due to a narrowed anoplasty. If the patient is remote and cannot easily come in for a clinic visit, have the family send a photo next to a coin. A dime (USA currency) is a size 14 Hegar. In the cases shown in Figure 25.8, the anoplasty on the left is adequately sized, but the anoplasty on the right has clearly narrowed and will need dilations or a revision.

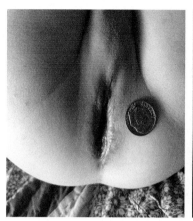 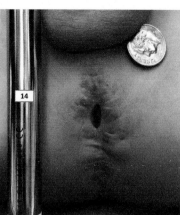

Figure 25.8 Photo of a coin next to an anoplasty to help determine if an anal stricture has developed.

MYTH: ROUTINE ANAL DILATIONS ARE NEEDED FOLLOWING PSARP TO PREVENT STRICTURES

Routine dilations are not necessary as they do not reduce stricture formation following PSARP. A recent single-institution, randomized, controlled clinical trial was conducted to evaluate the effect of dilation compared with non-dilation following PSARP for the primary outcome of stricture formation. An equal percentage of patients developed strictures, regardless of dilation (dilation 21%, non-dilation 32%, $p = 0.21$).

An HM anoplasty, a minor procedure, can be performed to manage a stricture if one develops. Non-dilation and an HM anoplasty, if needed, is a nice sequence to offer a family after PSARP rather than daily dilations. If a colostomy is in place, the HM anoplasty could be done at the same time as the stoma closure.

The HM anoplasty technique, described previously (Figure 24.5), makes a radial incision followed by longitudinal closure, which can convert a size 8 Hegar stricture to a size 16. However, this only works if the stricture is at skin level.

RECOMMENDED READING

Ahmad H, Skeritt C, Halleran DR, et al. Are routine postoperative dilations necessary after primary posterior sagittal anorectoplasty? A randomized controlled trial. *J Pediatr Surg*. 2021 Aug; 56(8): 1449–1453.

VAGINA PULLED THROUGH FOR THE ANOPLASTY

A 10-month-old female was referred for a severe stricture of the "anoplasty" after a PSARP for what was described as a short channel cloaca. Only a PSARP had been done, without any surgery on the urethra or vagina. On examination, you find a slightly recessed urethra that is otherwise normal. There is no vagina visible on a cystoscopic investigation, just a good length urethra, a normal bladder neck, and a normal bladder. The "anoplasty" is severely strictured. A contrast study was performed (Figure 25.9).

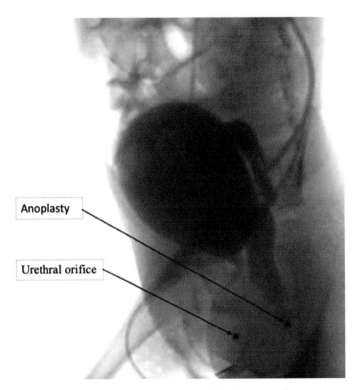

Figure 25.9 Initial contrast study, marked incorrectly.

What is the cause of the current condition?
What is your treatment plan?

The original surgery only involved what was thought to be the distal rectum, and the urethra and vagina supposedly were not touched. The contrast study reveals that, in fact, it was the vagina that was pulled through to the anoplasty during the prior operation, and a high distal rectum with a rectovaginal fistula was never recognized.

Laparoscopic mobilization of the high rectum was performed, dissecting the fistula but leaving it attached to the vagina. Then the patient was placed in prone position and the "anoplasty" was mobilized via a posterior sagittal incision, placing it at the introitus. This mobilized structure was, in fact, the native vagina (Figure 25.10). And, the mobilized distal rectum was placed at the anoplasty.

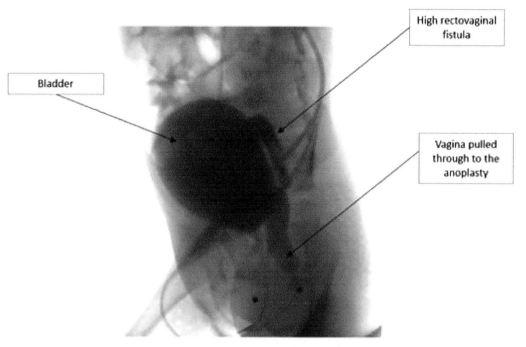

Figure 25.10 Contrast study, now labelled with actual anatomy encountered.

Surgeons work between the destiny of God and God's mercy.

**– Contributed by:
Mohamed Abdelmalak**

RECOMMENDED READING

Jocobs S, Tiusaba L, Bokova E, Al-Shamaileh T, Russell T, Varda B, Feng C, Badillo A, Levitt M. Where Is the Vagina? A Rectal Stricture after a Presumed Cloacal Repair Turns out to Be the Mobilized Vagina and a Missed High Rectovaginal Fistula. *European J Pediatr Surg Rep.* [In Press]

CHAPTER 26

PROBLEMS AFTER AN HD PULL-THROUGH

EVALUATION AND MANAGEMENT OF A HIRSCHSPRUNG DISEASE PATIENT WHO HAS HAD A PULL-THROUGH BUT IS NOT DOING WELL

In a patient who is not doing as expected following an HD pull-through, the surgeon should start by assessing into which category the patient's symptoms fall: obstructive symptoms or fecal soiling (Figure 26.1).

> Disease doesn't know boundaries and neither does talent.
>
> **– Contributed by: Julie Choueiki**

Obstructive symptoms: Symptoms of patients with obstruction can take various forms and include failure to thrive, recurrent episodes of enterocolitis, chronic abdominal distension, or a long-standing history of severe constipation that is refractory to medical management. These patients should be evaluated first with a contrast enema, followed by an EUA with rectal biopsy to look for a transition zone. At the time of EUA, the surgeon is looking at the anatomy to make sure that the dentate line is intact and the sphincters appear normal and are not patulous. These findings allow the surgeon to predict the patient's continence potential. The pathology of the biopsy should also return normal, meaning the presence of ganglion cells, the absence of hypertrophic nerves (less than 40 μm), and with a positive calretinin stain to indicate that there is not a transition zone. If the contrast enema or the EUA shows an abnormality, then the patient may need a redo pull-through for reasons such as stricture, retained Soave cuff, twist, Duhamel pouch, and transition zone. If the continence mechanism is deficient, with loss of the dentate line or overstretched sphincters, the surgeon should also consider a Malone placement at the time of the redo pull-through and/or spincter reconstruction. The goals of the redo are to both solve the obstruction and help the patient to be clean.

Suppose the anatomy, pathology, and contrast enema do not show any abnormalities that would warrant a reoperation. In that case, the surgeon should evaluate the sphincters for any dysfunction and determine if a trial of botulinum toxin would improve the obstructive symptoms. If there is no sphincter dysfunction, then the patient should start a bowel management program with optimization of either medical (laxatives) or mechanical (enemas or flushes) treatment.

Fecal soiling: For patients who have symptoms of fecal soiling, without a history of constipation or any obstruction, the physician can start the evaluation with a contrast enema and an EUA with 3D AMAN to evaluate the sphincter function. In cases of fecal soiling with no obstructive symptoms, the patient does not need a biopsy, as there is unlikely to be a transition zone since there is no obstruction. At the time of EUA, the surgeon should evaluate for an intact dentate line and good sphincter function. If these are normal, the patient should have bowel management for fecal soiling with medication to either slow down or speed up the stool, depending on the contrast study and whether the patient has hypomotility or hypermotility. If the EUA or 3D AMAN is abnormal, the surgeon could consider a procedure for sphincter reconstruction and/or a Malone to provide mechanical colonic emptying perhaps used as a bridge for future optimization of bowel control.

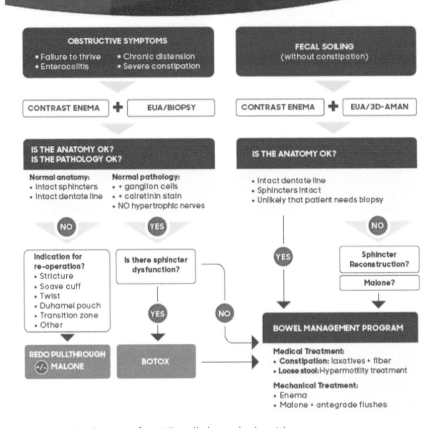

Figure 26.1 Evaluation after HD pull-through algorithm.

RECOMMENDED READING

Ahmad H, Yacob D, Halleran DR, Gasior AC, Di Lorenzo C, Wood RJ, Langer JC, Levitt MA. Evaluation and treatment of the post pull-through Hirschsprung patient who is not doing well, update for 2022. *Semin Pediatr Surg.* 2022; 31(2): 151164.

Langer JC. Persistent obstructive symptoms after surgery for Hirschsprung's disease: Development of a diagnostic and therapeutic algorithm. *J Pediatr Surg.* 2004 Oct; 39(10): 1458–1462.

Langer JC, Rollins MD, Levitt M, et al. Guidelines for the management of postoperative obstructive symptoms in children with Hirschsprung disease. *J Pediatr Surg.* 2017 May; 33(5): 523–526.

Levitt MA, Dickie B, Pena A. Evaluation and treatment of the patient with Hirschsprung disease who is not doing well after a pull-through procedure. *Semin Pediatr Surg.* 2010 May; 19(2): 146–153.

Levitt MA, Dickie B, Pena A. The Hirschsprungs patient who is soiling after what was considered a "successful" pull-through. *Semin Pediatr Surg.* 2012 Nov; 21(4): 344–353.

Levitt MA, Martin CA, Olesevich M, Bauer CL, Jackson LE, Pena A. Hirschsprung disease and fecal incontinence: Diagnostic and management strategies. *J Pediatr Surg.* 2009 Jan; 44(1): 271–277.

MYTH: PATIENTS WITH HIRSCHSPRUNG DISEASE WITHOUT A DENTATE LINE CANNOT ACHIEVE FECAL CONTINENCE

A damaged anal canal is a devastating complication of a pull-through procedure for HD, resulting in fecal incontinence. It occurs if the surgeon starts the pull-through too low and inadvertently excises the anal canal. Sphincters are required for tone around the pull-through (internal sphincter) and to voluntarily close the neorectum to hold stool to be released at the appropriate time (external sphincter). The sphincters can be overstretched during the transanal portion of the pull-through and thus permanently damaged. On examination of a patient with soiling, you find that the anal area demonstrates no dentate line, and, even when the patient is awake, the sphincters are patulous (Figure 26.2). These finding make fecal incontinence likely.

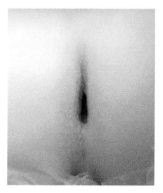

Figure 26.2

If there is an absent dentate line but the sphincters work, such a patient can achieve bowel control if they can detect stretch at the neorectum and close their voluntary sphincters in time.

There is no way to repair or replace a lost dentate line, but a sphincter-tightening surgical procedure can be a beneficial maneuver for patients suffering from true fecal incontinence due to patulous sphincters following a pull-through for HD.

In a sphincter reconstruction procedure, following circular mobilization of the very distal (3 cm) pull-through, the sphincter repair is initiated, placing several sutures in the anterior and posterior parts of the external sphincter muscle around the anal canal and attached to the pull-through (Figure 26.3).

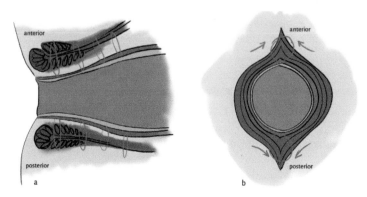

Figure 26.3

This sphincter tightening technique utilizes long-term absorbable sutures placed circumferentially around the external sphincter muscle and tacked to the pull-through to create a new closed anus surrounded by sphincters (Figures 26.4 and 26.5).

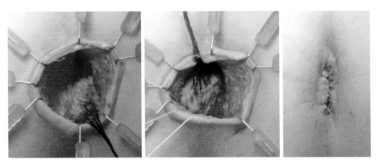

Figure 26.4 Sphincter-tightening procedure.

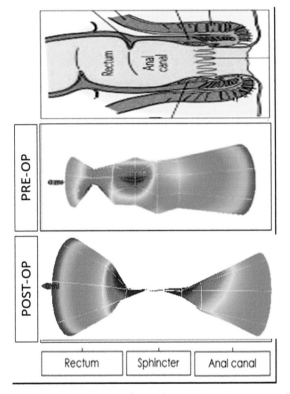

Figure 26.5 3D AMAN prior to and 1 month after sphincter reconstruction showing the inability of the sphincter to close the anal canal preoperatively but now able to do so postoperatively.

RECOMMENDED READING

Bokova E, McKenna E, Krois W, Reck CA, Al-Shamaileh T, Jacobs SE, Tiusaba L, Russell TL, Darbari A, Feng C, Badillo AT, Levitt ML. Reconstructing the Anal Sphincters to Reverse Iatrogenic Overstretching Following a Pull-through for Hirschsprung Disease. *J Pediatr Surg.* [In Press]

Krois W, Reck CA, Darbari A, Badillo A, Levitt MA. A technique to reconstruct the anal sphincters following iatrogenic stretching related to a pull-through for Hirschsprung disease. *J Pediatr Surg.* 2021; 56(6): 1242–1246.

CHRONIC CONSTIPATION AFTER A PULL-THROUGH

A 9-year-old patient had a prior transanal pull-through for HD at 1 month of age. The child presented with chronic constipation and daily soiling, but without enterocolitis episodes or failure to thrive. The contrast study is shown in Figure 26.6.

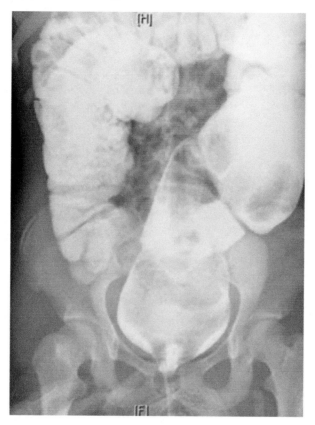

Figure 26.6 Contrast study.

A repeat rectal biopsy shows occasional ganglion cells and nerves measuring 50 μm. The dentate line and sphincters are preserved.

What is your treatment plan for this patient?

Just like in a patient with functional constipation, a patient with HD after pull-through can also have severe constipation and have ganglion cells and hypertrophic nerves on biopsy. According to the biopsy results, the patient is unlikely to have a transition zone pull-through because there are ganglion cells present. The mildly hypertrophic nerves are probably acquired from poor emptying, either because of non-relaxing sphincters or a dilated segment of colon. This can result from a lack of proactive treatment following an HD pull-through; ensuring good emptying with laxative and botulinum treatments of the nonrelaxing sphincters.

Medical treatment with laxatives, botulinum toxin injections, rectal enemas, or Malone antegrade continence enemas should be effective in this case.

> Tie your knots with love not passion.
>
> **– Robert Sawin**

However, non-relaxing sphincters may not let the antegrade flushes pass through and botulinum toxin to the sphincters might be needed (Figure 26.7). A redo of the primary surgery is not needed for a patient with such minimal obstructive symptoms.

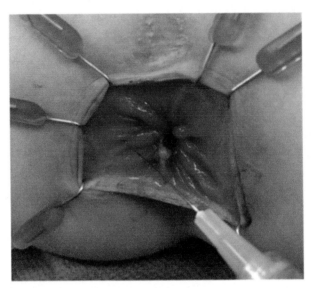

100 UI in 1 mL saline
4/8 positions

Figure 26.7 Botulinum toxin injection of the internal and external sphincters.

PATIENT POST-HD PULL-THROUGH WITH FECAL SOILING AND A DISTENDED COLON

A 5-year-old girl who had a newborn HD pull-through has done well over the years. She now presents at school age with soiling, having four or five loose stools per day. She has normal height and weight, no abdominal distension, and has never suffered from enterocolitis. Her contrast study is shown in Figure 26.8.

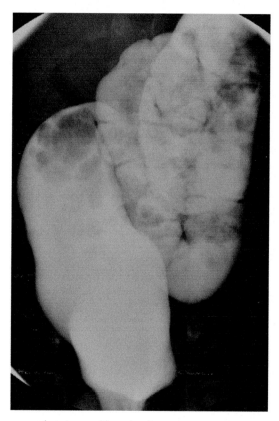

Figure 26.8 Contrast enema showing a dilated colon.

What would be your plan for evaluation and likely treatment?

The contrast enema shows a dilated colon impacted with stool. If the sphincters are not relaxing, the 4–5 stools are probably related to overflow, just like in a patient with functional constipation. A stricture, cuff, or twist must be ruled out. She may need botulinum toxin injections to help her learn to overcome her sphincter non-relaxation. She most likely needs laxatives to provoke the colon to empty (provided her dentate line and sphincters are intact).

In this case, a clean out should be performed first, followed by daily senna administration. The senna is needed to empty the colon each day, and the addition of water-soluble fiber helps to provide bulk to the stool. Once she is able to have one to two well-formed stools per day and is emptying the colon well, she should have bowel control.

PATIENT POST-HD PULL-THROUGH WITH FECAL SOILING AND A NON-DISTENDED COLON

Another 5-year-old girl with an HD pull-through as a newborn presents to clinic at school age with soiling. She is having four or five loose stools per day. She has a normal height and weight, no abdominal distension, and has never suffered from enterocolitis. Her contrast study is shown in Figure 26.9.

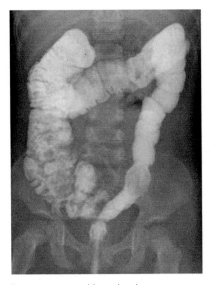

Figure 26.9 Contrast enema showing a nondilated colon.

What would be your plan for evaluation and likely treatment?

In a child with HD and a previous pull-through, a detailed evaluation of the history, the type of operation previously performed, EUA with biopsy, and a contrast enema should be performed. It is vitally important to treat the patient, not the X-ray.

This patient is stooling too much. Given her lack of obstructive symptoms, this child may be suffering from hypermotility, as the distal colon is not dilated. An EUA will help you assess the sphincters and the dentate line, and rule out a mechanical obstruction from a cuff, stricture, or retained aganglionosis. All are unlikely here, given the absence of obstructive symptoms.

If this same X-ray were present for a patient presenting with obstructive symptoms and episodes of enterocolitis, this could represent retained transition zone, which would require surgery.

But, in this case, with multiple stools a day, it represents a colon that moves too fast. If the EUA confirms a normal dentate line and normal sphincters, stool transit needs to be slowed down. The bowel movement pattern should be adjusted to strive for one to two well-formed stools per day. With that pattern, achieved with a constipating diet, some water-soluble fiber, and some loperamide, this patient was able to have bowel control within 1 week.

The patient's ability to have voluntary bowel movements will depend on the original surgery's success in preserving her sphincters and dentate line. If both are absent, then bowel management with enemas or a Malone would be the treatment.

CHAPTER 27

DECIDING WHEN TO DO A REDO PROCEDURE IN HD

POST-HIRSCHSPRUNG DISEASE PULL-THROUGH WITH OBSTRUCTIVE SYMPTOMS

A 2-year-old boy with a prior laparoscopic-assisted Soave pull-through for HD has had four admissions for enterocolitis. A digital rectal exam did not show an anastomotic stricture. Botulinum toxin injections helped to improve the condition for about 1 month each time, but then obstructive symptoms recurred. The contrast study is shown in Figure 27.1.

> Since light travels faster than sound, some people appear bright until you hear them speak.
>
> **– Contributed by: Marc Levitt**

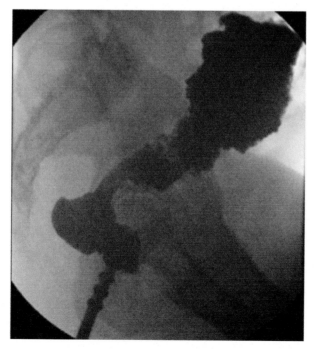

Figure 27.1 Contract enema showing a circumferential narrowing of the distal pull-through.

What is causing the symptoms?

The contrast study reveals an obstructive Soave cuff looking like a Nissen fundoplication around the pull-through. Note the enlarged presacral space. The cuff probably rolled up or was cut but incompletely divided. Either way, it is causing a ring-like constriction of the pull-through and should be palpable on digital exam. The cuff is the original outer wall of the rectum and is aganglionic thus causing a functional obstruction.

DOI: 10.1201/9781003150015-31

> You should 'own' problems you are presented with before making 'your problems' someone else's problem'.
>
> **– Contributed by: Megan Durham**

Removal of the cuff is recommended. A transanal dissection of the distal pull-through found the cuff surrounding the initial pull-through (Figure 27.2). In most cases, the transanal approach is preferable. However, sometimes the cuff is accessible through the abdomen in older versions of the Soave during which the cuff was started in the pelvis. The presence of ganglion cells in the distal pull-through also needs to be confirmed to rule out a transition zone pull-through.

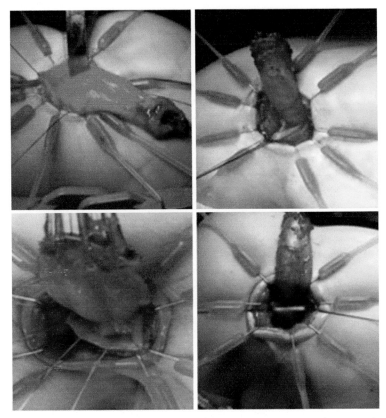

Figure 27.2 Four examples of retained Soave cuff excision via a transanal approach.

RETAINED TRANSITION ZONE

The contrast enema shown in Figure 27.3 represents a concern for a transition zone pull-through. If you see this finding in a patient with obstructive symptoms, you can predict the likelihood of a retained transition zone. Note this distal segment is ahaustral, without peristalsis. The rectum is similar in shape to a summer squash. Of course, a biopsy must be performed to confirm your suspicion, which may show the absence of ganglion cells and the presence of nerves greater than 40 µm.

> Common sense is anything but common.
>
> **– Mark Twain**

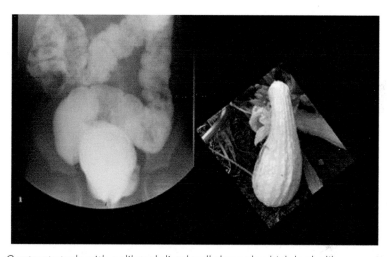

Figure 27.3 Contrast study with a dilated distal pull-through which looks like a summer squash.

A PROBLEMATIC DUHAMEL PULL-THROUGH

More is missed by not seeing than by not knowing.

– Alberto Peña

A 2-year-old child with total colonic HD underwent an ileo-Duhamel pull-through at 10 months. Over the last year, the patient has presented with enterocolitis four times. A contrast enema is shown in Figure 27.4.

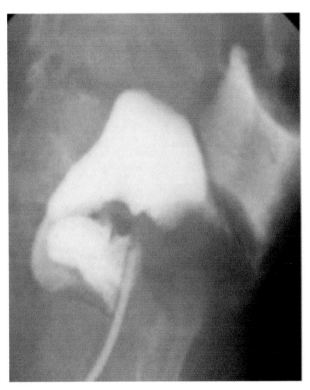

Figure 27.4 Contrast study following an ileo-Duhamel pull-through.

Is there a problem with the pull-through? If so, how would you fix it?

In this patient, there is a spur where the Duhamel pouch and the pulled-through ileum were not adequately united into a single lumen at the original operation. One can see two separate lumens in the pelvis. The pouch fills with stool and then obstructs the proximal ileum by pressing it against the sacrum. The treatment is to remove the spur with a stapler transanally (see Figure 27.5). If it is not possible to do this or if removal of the common wall (spur) does not improve the symptoms, a redo ileoanal pull-through with removal of the Duhamel pouch is needed.

A colo-Duhamel is shown in Figure 27.6. Again, there is inadequate mating of the two lumens – the so-called "spur" – and this problem can be fixed in the same way. Sometimes, the pouch itself

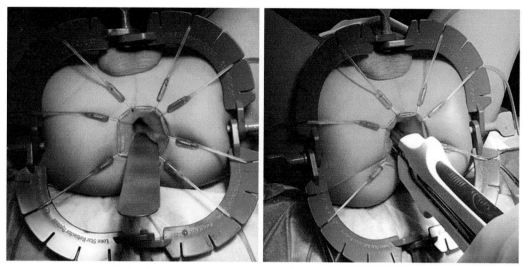

Figure 27.5 Duhamel spur removal using stapler. An endovasular stapler can also be used.

imposes too much stasis on the ganglionated part of the pull-through and must be removed. An ideal pouch is one that is short, below the peritoneal reflection, and fully mated to unite the native rectum and the pull-through.

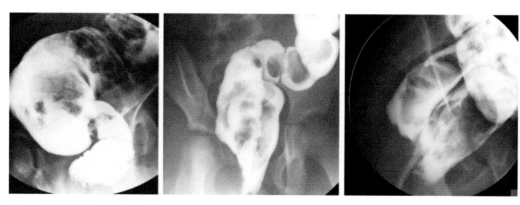

Figure 27.6 Colo-Duhamel.

POST-SOAVE PULL-THROUGH WITH RECURRENT ENTEROCOLITIS

A 7-year-old child who underwent a Soave pull-through in the newborn period presents with significant obstructive symptoms, multiple episodes of enterocolitis, and regular bloating, which are somewhat responsive to irrigations. His contrast enema can be seen in Figure 27.7.

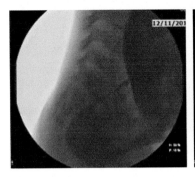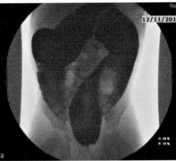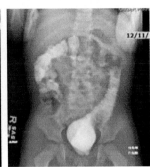

Figure 27.7

> There are lots of ways to make a simple operation hard.
>
> **– Fred Ryckman**

What do you notice about the contrast study? What would you recommend for treatment?

The distal portion of the pull-through is dilated, and particularly the neorectum is ahaustral and inert (most visible on the post-evacuation film). The mucosa of the left colon appears to be irregular, consistent with a low-grade enterocolitis. The distal segment is concerning for a transition zone pull-through (summer squash appearance), and the biopsy confirmed that there were no ganglion cells. This patient subsequently underwent a removal of that segment and had a pull-through of the left colon which contained good ganglion cells and normal-size nerves. The patient now is stooling without difficulty.

What would you do for a workup? If you did a colonic motility evaluation, what is it likely to show?

There is no need to do a colonic motility study until you have evaluated for a distal obstruction. If such a study were to be done prior to evaluating for a distal obstruction, it may show that the entire colon is dysmotile, leading a surgeon to perform a colon resection, which would be the wrong thing to do. The colon is actually in proper condition, and the distal pull-through is the problem. So, the lesson here is to rule out a distal problem. Is it a stricture, a cuff, a twist, or a transition zone pull-through? If none of the above problems exists, then it is likely the non-relaxing internal sphincter causing obstructive symptoms, and this can be solved with botulinum toxin injection.

PART V
MISCELLANEOUS COLORECTAL TOPICS AND TECHNIQUES

CHAPTER 28

OPERATING ROOM SETUP AND POSITIONING

OPERATING ROOM SETUP: TOTAL BODY PREP

When perineal and abdominal approaches may be needed, utilizing a total body prep saves operative time and facilitates surgical decision-making by having ready access to both surgical fields. Only one set of instruments is required.

The process of a total body prep, which allows the surgeon to perform part of the procedure prone, turn the patient while under the sterile drapes, and continue the operation in a supine position via the abdomen, is shown in the series of photos in Figure 28.1.

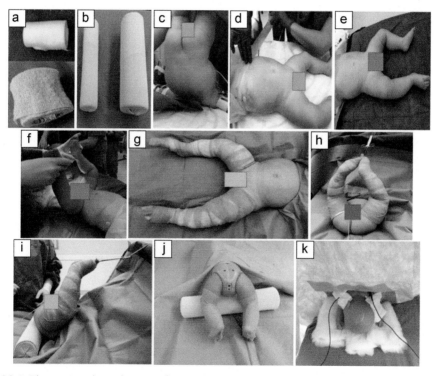

Figure 28.1 The materials and steps of a sterile total body prep are shown. (a) Webril and Coban. (b) Sterile rolls. (c) Placing cautery pad. (d), (e) Lower body is prepped. (f) Legs are elevated for prep. (g) Lower body now circumferentially prepped. (h) Front view and (i) side view of legs secured in an elevated position for supine transanal approach. (j) Prone position of total body prep. (k) Cushioning of head in prone position.

The cautery pad is placed high on the back, with two 1000 drapes encircling the patient prior to prepping, so the pad does not get wet. After prepping, soft sterile Webril wrap and then Coban are used to wrap the lower extremities. Sterile rolls are placed under the hips. The patient is placed following sterile preparation through the circular opening of the surgical extremity drape.

DOI: 10.1201/9781003150015-33

OPERATING ROOM SETUP: PRONE POSITIONING

When in doubt, mumble.

– Contributed by: Michael Phillips

Prone positioning is shown in Figure 28.2. Proper padding is needed under pressure points. Be sure to support the ankles and hips. Insert a cushion under the head and axillae to protect the airway and endotracheal tube and avoid hyperextension of the neck and shoulders (Figure 28.3). The pelvis should be tilted, with the buttocks higher than the chest to optimize exposure.

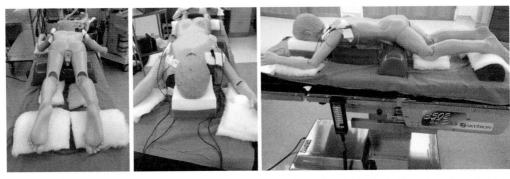

Figure 28.2 A patient in prone position is shown, with cushioning of the head and neck highlighted in middle picture and padding of pressure points in the right picture.

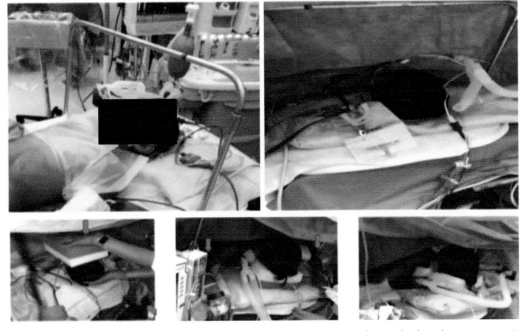

Figure 28.3 The top left picture shows the ether screen, and right shows the head in prone position. The bottom row of pictures highlights the protection of the head, neck, endotracheal tube, and axillae.

HOW TO SEE IN THE DARK: DEEP PELVIC DISSECTION

When dissecting deep in the pelvis, especially for older patients, it is sometimes hard to see. The lighted St. Marks retractor (Figure 28.4) is a handy tool as it allows for retraction of deep pelvic structures while incorporating a light source.

Pressure makes diamonds.

– Dominic Purpura, medical school dean, to Marc Levitt when he was a brand new medical student

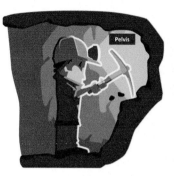
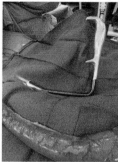
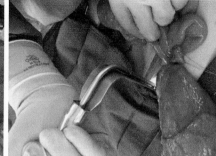

Figure 28.4 Lighting for the deep pelvis.

MOBILIZATION OF STRUCTURES: CIRCUMFERENTIAL TENSION

To mobilize structures such as during the transanal dissection, placing multiple silk sutures allows the surgeon to provide circumferential tension and helps to visualize the dissection plane (Figure 28.5). Place more sutures, not fewer, to provide equal tension, and use the sutures to remove folds in the mucosa.

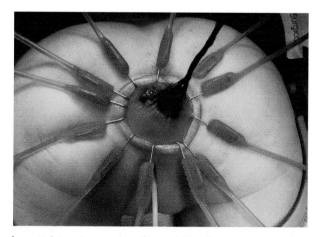

Figure 28.5 Circumferential traction sutures for mobilization.

SURGICAL EXPOSURE

Adequate surgical field exposure is a principle in all surgeries, and, in colorectal surgery, this has been improved significantly by using a lone star retractor and its pins (Figure 28.6). However, if you do not have a lone star retractor, adequate exposure can be attained using self-retaining retractors, sutures, and skin hooks secured to the drapes. Be sure that your drapes are held firmly in place by suturing them to the patient if you do not have adhesive drapes.

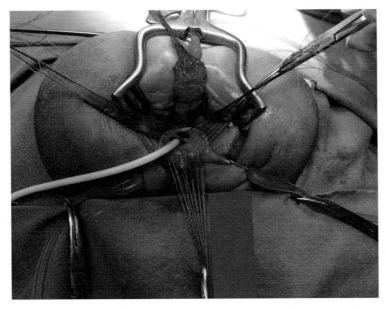

Figure 28.6 Perineal exposure.

MULTI-TASKING LONE STAR PINS

Lone star pins were originally used to facilitate the transanal dissection for HD cases (Figure 28.7). However, they can also be used to provide exposure during a PSARP. The pins apply uniform, circumferential tension to the sides of the incision and are particularly useful when a Weitlaner retractor is too large to fit the incision. You can use the lone star ring or just clip the pins to the drapes, ensuring the drapes are held firmly to the patient.

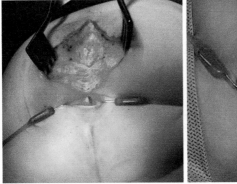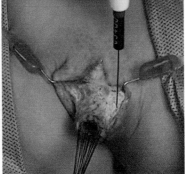

Figure 28.7 Lone star pins used for exposure.

BOWEL PREPARATION

A bowel prep is needed for all patients undergoing a PSARP or redo PSARP without a diverting ostomy, for patients with cloaca if a vaginal replacement might be needed, for patients with functional constipation who are undergoing a colonic resection, for patients with HD

> It's less about learning new things and more about letting go of old things.
>
> – Liza Miller

without a diverting ostomy or who need their ostomy pulled through, or for patients undergoing a neo-Malone procedure (Figure 28.8).

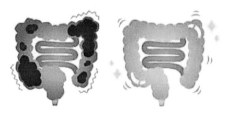

- ✓ PSARP with no ostomy
- ✓ Anticipation of vaginal replacement
- ✓ Sigmoid resection (2 days)
- ✓ HD no ostomy
- ✓ Redo HD/PSARP
- ✓ Neomalone

Figure 28.8 Bowel prep indications.

Combined preoperative mechanical bowel preparation with oral antibiotics significantly reduces rates of surgical site infection, anastomotic leak, and ileus after colorectal surgery.

Start clear liquids/Pedialyte on the day of the bowel prep, usually 24 hours before surgery, except for those undergoing colon resection due to colonic dysmotility. For those, this should be started 48 hours prior to surgery.

The patient is given PEG 3350 (Golytely), an osmotic laxative with electrolytes at a rate of 25 mL/kg/hr × 4 hours. For babies, an NG tube is placed, and for older kids who can tolerate that amount of liquids, this can be given by mouth. The prep can also be run through a Malone or cecostomy or a gastrostomy tube if one is present. Additionally, peripheral intravenous (IV) access to administer maintenance fluids adjusted by weight is required for hydration.

To improve colonic emptying, rectal irrigations may be needed, particularly in HD patients. When used, irrigations are initiated at the start of the preparation with normal saline to help evacuate the stools. The patient is irrigated with saline every 2 hours, 10–20 mL at a time, until clear (max volume to retain is 20 mL/kg).

The oral antibiotics Neomycin and Erythromycin are given 1, 2, and 4 hours after stool output is clear and Golytely is complete. The patient is made NPO (nil per os) at midnight the night before surgery but clear liquids can be continued until 2 hours before surgery (Figure 28.9). Remember to stop the oral preparation in time for the anesthetic NPO requirement.

- Clear liquids/Pedialyte on day of bowel prep
- Golytely (25 mL/kg/hr)
  - Max dose: 500 mL/hr
  - PO, NG, GT, Malone, cecostomy
- Rectal irrigations
- IV access, maintenance IV fluids
- Blood work: Glucose, Ca$^+$, Na$^+$, K$^+$, CO_2, Chloride, BUN, Creatinine, and CBC
- Neomycin and Metronidazole x 3 doses: Give at 1, 2, and 4 hr
- NPO at Midnight, clear liquids until 2 hours prior to surgery

Figure 28.9

ANAL DILATIONS

Good judgment comes from bad experiences, which comes from bad judgment.

— **Arthur Aufses**

Rectal dilations are an intervention to keep an anal opening patent enough to be able to pass stool effectively (Figure 28.10). Patients who need rectal dilations are most commonly those with ARMs, sometimes post HD pull-through patients, and patients who develop an anal stricture after surgery. Dilation schedules vary depending on the timeline – preoperative or postoperative. If prescribed for a patient prior to surgery, dilations should happen through the rectoperineal or vestibular fistula twice a day, each day until surgery, using a size that is comfortable yet large enough to allow stool to pass. After surgery, if a stricture is developing, dilations will initially start 2 to 4 weeks postoperatively. They should be done twice daily, increasing by one dilator size until the goal size is reached. Prophylactic dilations are not routinely necessary because they are not any better than not dilating to avoid a stricture after PSARP, as has been shown by a recent randomized controlled trial. If dilations are needed to treat a stricture, the surgeon will determine the appropriate starting size of dilator that inserts comfortably into the neoanus or pull-through neorectum. The designated dilator goal size is determined based upon age. Once dilations reach the appropriate goal size, dilations can be tapered in frequency over the next several months.

With the increasing size of dilators, it is typical to have streaks of blood on the dilator owing to the stretching of the anal canal. Blood streaks are expected and should not cause discontinuation of the dilations. The larger size dilator may also be challenging to pass. Should this occur, try using more lubricant, giving a gentle twist or spin of the dilator when inserting, warming the dilator, or using a smaller size dilator immediately followed by the larger dilator.

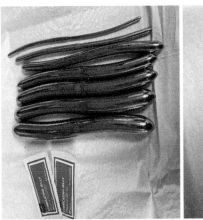 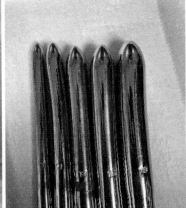

Figure 28.10 Anal dilators.

The most used dilators to check or dilate the anoplasty after a PSARP or the colo-anal anastomosis after an HD pull-through are sizes 11–14. If Hegar dilators cannot be obtained, substitutes for the most common sizes are easy to find. Examples of substitutes include the top cap of an enema bottle, a 5 mL blood collection tube, graded candles, a 3D printed model, and the caregiver's gloved little finger (Figure 28.11).

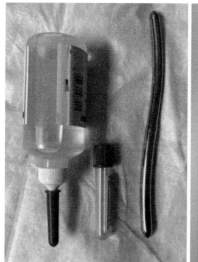 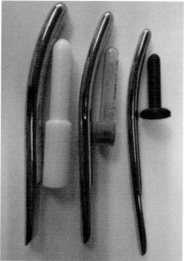

Figure 28.11 Alternatives for anal dilation.

The oak gets strong in the storm.
(translated from German)

– Contributed by: Martin Lacher

RECOMMENDED READING

Ahmad H, Skeritt C, Halleran DR, et al. Are routine postoperative dilations necessary after primary posterior sagittal anorectoplasty? A randomized controlled trial. *J Pediatr Surg.* 2021 Aug; 56(8): 1449–1453.

ULTRASOUND-GUIDED BOTULINUM TOXIN INJECTION

Using a hockey stick ultrasound probe, one can display the external sphincter and the deeper thickening of the internal sphincter's circular muscular layer. Placing the probe in the longitudinal axis allows the operator to follow the percutaneously punctured needle and position the tip exactly in the internal sphincter (shown in Figures 28.12 and 28.13).

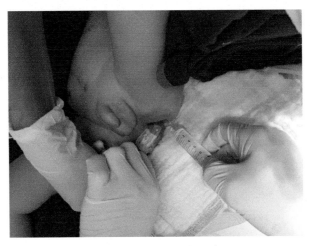

Figure 28.12 Injecting botulinum toxin with ultrasound guidance.

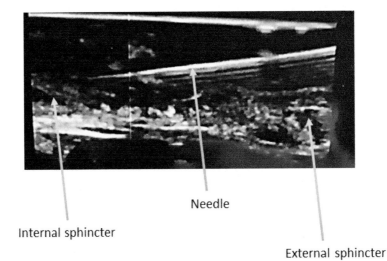

Needle

Internal sphincter

External sphincter

Figure 28.13 Ultrasound showing the internal and external sphincters and the needle.

RECOMMENDED READING

Church JT, Gadepalli SK, Talishinsky T, Teitelbaum DH, Jarboe MD. Ultrasound-guided intrasphincteric botulinum toxin injection relieves obstructive defecation due to Hirschsprung's disease and internal anal sphincter achalasia. *J Pediatr Surg*. 2017; 52: 74–78.

SUBTLE DISSECTION WITH ELECTROCAUTERY

Decreasing the settings of the electrocautery to as low as possible enables the surgeon to use this tool for very subtle dissection. It does not cut through the tissue layers but allows the surgeon to find the planes separating the layers. Figure 28.14 shows the dissection of the thin vaginal wall off the rectum in a rare case of an ARM with a rectovaginal fistula.

> The only way to a wicked man's heart is through surgery.
>
> **– Contributed by: Bu Nguyen**

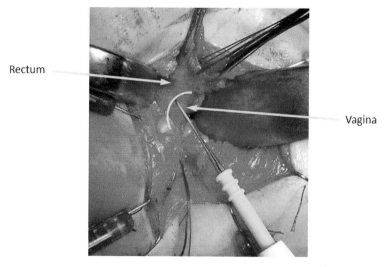

Figure 28.14 Subtle electrocautery dissection using low settings.

Chapter 29

STOMAS

TAPERING TO MAKE THE STOMA A MORE REASONABLE SIZE

Tapering the stoma is a nice trick you can use when creating any kind of stoma (ileostomy or colostomy) if the piece of bowel is too wide. After stapling or oversewing the bowel segment, take the corner and remove the cone (Figure 29.1). The size of the cone should be based on the size of the stoma that you desire. The staple line can be imbricated. Over time, the dilated bowel proximal to the stoma will decompress.

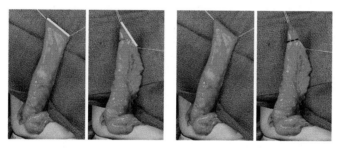

Figure 29.1 Tapering the stoma for the desired circle size.

ANASTOMOSIS WITH LARGE SIZE DISCREPANCY

Large size discrepancies may occur with small bowel or colonic atresia or, rarely, for a colostomy closure. When one needs to perform an anastomosis with a large size discrepancy, one nice trick is to create a proximal "blow hole" to protect the anastomosis.

In Figure 29.2, you see an almost 10:1 size difference and, essentially, an end to side anastomosis, which is precarious. Opening a small stoma just proximal to the anastomosis on the anti-mesenteric side of the bowel allows for some stool to exit the stoma and some to go through the anastomosis. Over time, the distal segment will grow and accept more pressure and stool. Then, the "blow hole" stoma can be closed.

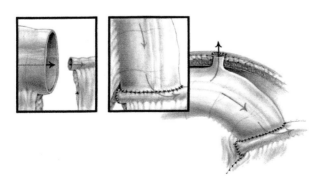

Figure 29.2 Blow hole to protect an anastomosis with a significant size discrepancy.

DOI: 10.1201/9781003150015-34

CLOSING THE MUCUS FISTULA TO AVOID SPILLAGE

When the going gets tough at a particular area of dissection, let's just go somewhere else.

– Contributed by: Alp Numanglo

In the case of the loop stoma, when you wish to avoid distal spillage, simply pursestring close the distal segment (Figure 29.3). This prevents stool from crossing to the distal segment. Before closing the distal segment in this way, make sure that stool has been evacuated through irrigation.

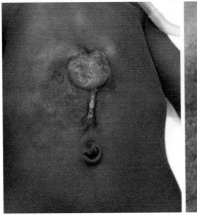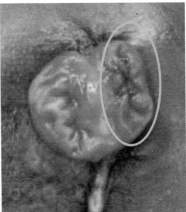

Figure 29.3 Pursestring closure of the distal part of a loop stoma to prevent stool spillage across.

CREATING A STOMA AND AVOIDING STOMAL PROLAPSE

There are two techniques to avoid stoma prolapse.

In the row of pictures in Figure 29.4, the bowel wall is tacked to the anterior abdominal wall, and the stoma comes out a separate opening. This tacking is used when you have an abdominal incision.

A part of good science is to see what everyone else can see but think what no one else has ever said.

– Contributed by: Amos Tversky

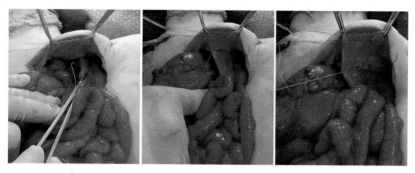

Figure 29.4 Preventing stoma prolapse if there is an abdominal incision.

In the rows of pictures in Figure 29.5, the bowel is tacked inside the circle made for the stoma creation when there is no other incision besides the stoma site. Place a clamp in one corner and hold it up, and then tack the bowel to the anterior abdominal wall. At the surface, the bowel will take a slight turn (illustrated by the pipe picture), which will help to prevent prolapse. This tack is for when you use laparascopy to create the stoma.

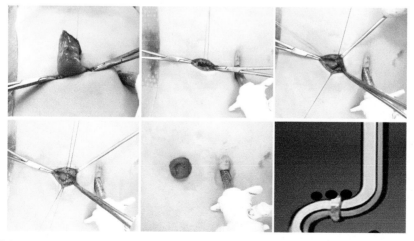

Figure 29.5 Preventing stoma prolapse if there is no incision other than the hole for the stoma.

TREATING A STOMAL PROLAPSE

To manage a stoma prolapse, a critical first move is to reduce the prolapse. Sometimes the stoma can be reduced by packing the stoma with betadine-soaked gauze. The gauze can grip the lumen and de-intussuscept it. Sometimes an incision must be made to reduce the prolapse.

Once the prolapse is reduced, you can then palpate that segment of the bowel through the abdominal wall and place a Hegar dilator into the lumen. Then, through a separate incision (if the patient has an abdominal scar that can be used) the abdomen is opened there, and the bowel wall can then be tacked to the anterior abdominal wall (Figure 29.6). This effectively prevents future prolapse and additionally avoids any dissection at the stoma site itself.

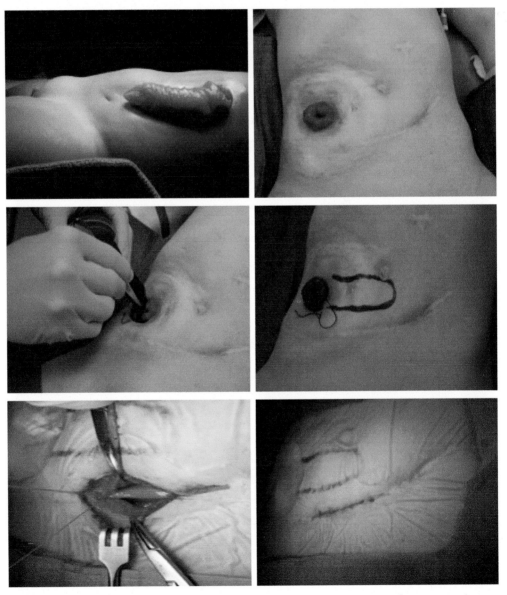

Figure 29.6 Tacking the bowel to the anterior abdominal wall to prevent a future re-prolapse.

TAKING DOWN A COLOSTOMY AND AVOIDING DOG EARS

When excising a colostomy site (or any circular area), if you excise an ellipse of tissue with a ratio of 3:1 relative to the diameter of the circle, at the end of the case there will not be dog ears, and the incision will close nicely as a straight line (Figure 29.7).

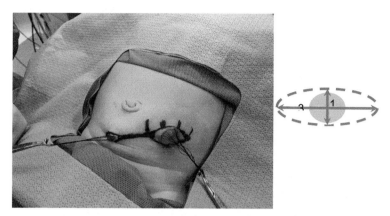

Figure 29.7 Closing a colostomy site to avoid dog ears.

When taking down a colostomy, circumferential silk sutures placed around the colostomy and mucus fistula provide excellent traction and control of the bowel (Figure 29.8).

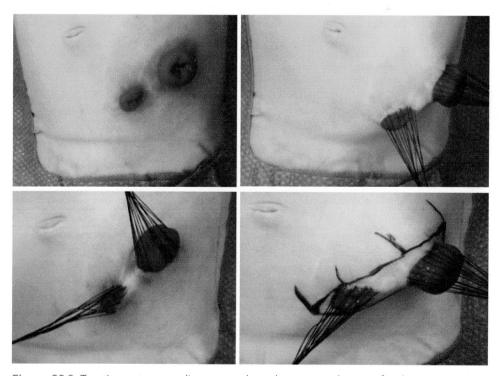

Figure 29.8 Traction sutures to dissect out the colostomy and mucus fistula.

CLOSING THE MESENTERIC DEFECT IN A STOMA CLOSURE

Nothing has ever been accomplished in any walk of life without enthusiasm, without motivation, and without perseverance.

– Jim Valvano

A nice way to close a mesenteric defect is to place a mosquito clamp onto the mesenteric fat on either side of the defect and place a tie at the bottom of the two clamps (Figures 29.9 and 29.10). This technique avoids possibly injuring the blood vessels if the surgeon attempts to close the defect using a suture.

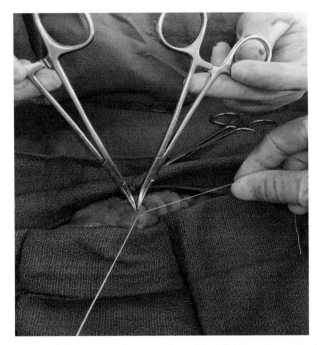

Figure 29.9 Two mosquito clamps grasp fat on either side of the mesenteric defect.

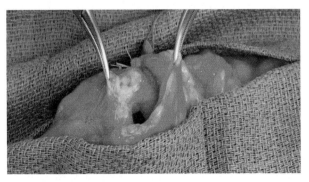

Figure 29.10 Close-up view.

TROUBLESHOOTING PERISTOMAL SKIN BREAKDOWN

In the event of peristomal breakdown, use the following questions to help troubleshoot and pinpoint the issue to aid in treatment (Figure 29.11).

1. Is the stoma flush to the skin or budded (raised above skin level)? If flush, is a flat or convex wafer being used?
2. Is the stoma in skin folds on the abdomen or the groin? If yes, is the Eakin seal being used to help fill in the hills and valleys to make a flat pouching surface?
3. Does the wafer need to go over the umbilical area? If yes, is a flexible pouch being used?
4. Does the stool come out of the middle of the stoma, or off to the side of the stoma? If the stoma is lying on the side and the stool is coming from the side, is a convex wafer being used?
5. How much stool is in the pouch when it is emptied? What is the consistency? If it is normally watery, has a PPI been used to help neutralize the stool pH?
6. Look at the back of the wafer before it is discarded. Has it been "eaten away" from the stool? See # 5 for intervention.
7. Does it appear to be yeasty and itchy around the stoma? If yes, try having the pouch changed daily, with Nystatin powder applied, and set with a barrier wipe. If no better in 24–48 hours, may need to be treated with a systemic antifungal.

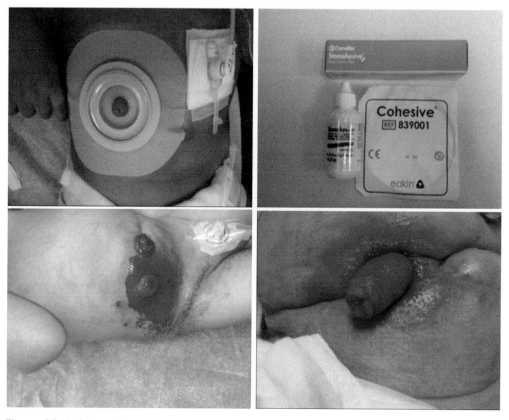

Figure 29.11 Stoma site care.

Pediatric Colorectal Surgery: Tips & Tricks

BAGGING OPTIONS FOR STOMAS

Bagging of stomas can be challenging in low-resource areas where there is the scarce availability of bags, adhesives, and support for families of children with stomas. This has led to some creative innovations, as seen in Figure 29.12.

A surgical glove has been folded around a plastic ring cut from a plastic container, held in place with a fabric band on the top. In the middle is a condom pulled through a hole cut into a sanitary towel. The adhesive on the sanitary towel helps hold this collection device in place. On the bottom, the simplest method is to "double diaper." The drawback to this method is the risk for excoriation of the surrounding skin if a sufficient amount of barrier cream is not applied.

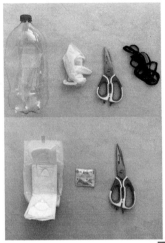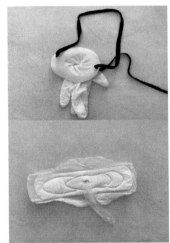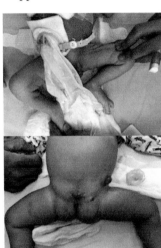

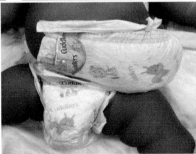

Figure 29.12 Innovative ways to bag a stoma.

CHAPTER 30

ISCHIORECTAL FAT PAD

ISCHIORECTAL FAT PAD (GONZALEZ HERNIA): PSARP VERSION

An ischiorectal fat pad is a great source of tissue to cover the posterior urethra or vagina if coverage is needed – for example, in a redo case. The ischiorectal fat is visible in the posterior sagittal incision, and it is grasped with a suture and pulled out (Figure 30.1). The fat remains pedicalized and then can cover the repair.

When doing a difficult operation always do the easier part first. You'll find that the harder part is then easier.

– Bernie Langer, hepatobiliary surgeon and father of Jack Langer

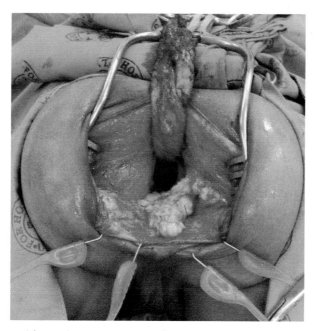

Figure 30.1 Ischiorectal fat pad, posterior sagittal incision.

DOI: 10.1201/9781003150015-35

ISCHIORECTAL FAT PAD (GONZALEZ HERNIA): TRANSANAL VERSION

The ischiorectal fat pad can also be used during a transanal approach (Figure 30.2). It is not as easy to find as it is with a posterior sagittal incision. You need to gently split the sphincter muscles on one of the lateral sides, and right behind these fibers is the ischiorectal space. The fat is grasped and mobilized to cover the space anteriorly, like for repair of an acquired rectovaginal fistula in HD.

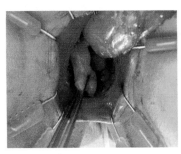 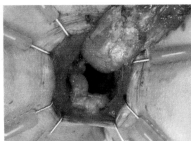

Figure 30.2 Ischiorectal fat accessed during a transanal incision.

RECOMMENDED READING

Levitt MA, King SK, Bischoff A, Alam S, Pena A. The Gonzalez hernia revisited: Use of the ischiorectal fat pad to aid in the repair of rectovaginal and rectourethral fistulae. *J Pediatr Surg.* 2014 Aug; 49(8): 1308–1310.

Tiusaba L, Jacobs SE, Al-Shamaileh T, Bokova E, Russell TL, Badillo AT, Feng C, Levitt MA. The Gonzalez Hernia (Ischiorectal Fat Pad) Occurring During a Posterior Sagittal Anorectoplasty (PSARP) – The Historical Context of a Technical Error That Led to a Helpful New Technique. *J Pediatr Surg.* [In Press]

CHAPTER 31

MISCELLANEOUS COLORECTAL CONDITIONS

NEWBORN INTESTINAL OBSTRUCTION: COLONIC ATRESIA

A newborn with intestinal obstruction is evaluated in the NICU. A presurgical contrast enema and the operative findings are presented in Figure 31.1. The anus is normal.

> There is no basement to stupidity.
>
> – **Michael Caty**

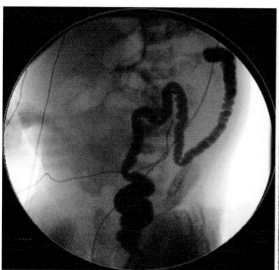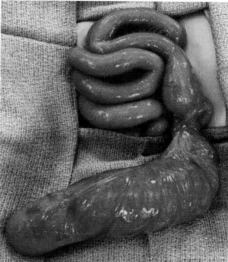

Figure 31.1 Contrast study and operative findings in a newborn with intestinal obstruction.

What would you do?

The newborn has colonic atresia. A rectal biopsy should be performed, given the association with HD, and an end colostomy with the end of the atresia created. The association is rare, but it is important to ensure that a future anastomosis will not result in distal obstruction from HD. If you have a good frozen section available to you, that is an option, but frozen section analysis may not be possible.

The results of the biopsy dictate operative considerations, as does the overall dilation of the bulbous end of the atresia. If the biopsy returns with HD, you can perform a pull-through of the stoma. If there is no HD, then you can reconstruct using a colo-colonic anastomosis (with or without tapering, depending on how much shrinking the colon does) or perform an ileocolic anastomosis with resection of the bulbous colon.

DOI: 10.1201/9781003150015-36

BILATERAL HYDRONEPHROSIS AND A PELVIC MASS

A full-term infant is born with prenatally diagnosed bilateral hydronephrosis and a pelvic mass. The perineal exam is shown in Figure 31.2.

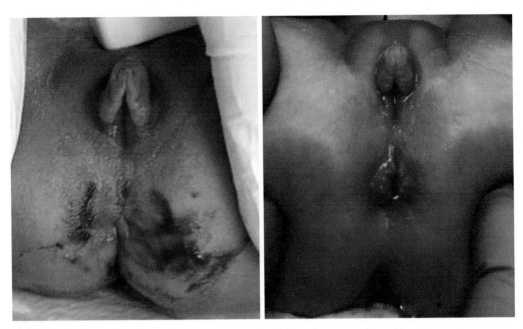

Figure 31.2 Perineum of an infant with bilateral hydronephrosis and a pelvic mass.

What type of malformation is this?

The first photo shows an anal opening that suggests a perineal fistula. However, the second photo is higher quality with better exposure and shows a normal and adequately sized anus. Given a normal anal opening, the malformation is consistent with a urogenital (UG) sinus instead of a cloaca. The pelvic mass is a hydrocolpos, which developed from urine passing into the vagina, and is causing the hydronephrosis.

What would you do to intervene?

To confirm the diagnosis and make a plan for surgical reconstruction, a cystoscopy and vaginoscopy should be performed. The cystoscopy and vaginoscopy provide information about the length of the common channel and the length of the urethra. The hydrocolpos can be drained through perineal catheterization. The ultimate repair should be guided by endoscopy and a contrast study (3D cloacagram). If the confluence of the UG sinus is high, an anterior sagittal transrectal approach (ASTRA) or transanorectal approach can be used to provide exposure and further assist in total urogenital mobilization. A very high UG confluence can be managed laparoscopically or robotically.

What would be your plan of care after the newborn period?

A key determinant in the plan of care is the severity of hydronephrosis. Severe hydronephrosis can lead to renal dysplasia and a poor renal prognosis. Additionally, it is important to figure out if this condition involves an adrenogenital syndrome.

SACRAL NERVE STIMULATION (SNS)

Sacral nerve stimulation (SNS) was originally designed to treat women after childbirth who suffered from urinary incontinence and an overactive bladder. It was soon discovered that it could be used to treat fecal incontinence as well.

Culture is what you do when no one's watching.

– Contributed by: Julie Choueiki

A potential population for use of SNS in children are patients with ARM with borderline continence potential. Another group are patients with severe functional constipation unresponsive to medical management. It has been used on this population with varying degrees of success in terms of fecal continence. It is very successful in managing urinary symptoms. The procedure consists of two phases, 1–2 weeks apart. In the first phase, the "test phase," the electrodes are hooked up to an external battery. If the patient has a 50% improvement of symptoms, then they may progress to the second phase or the more permanent implant (Figure 31.3).

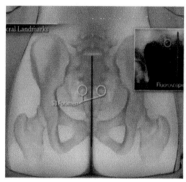
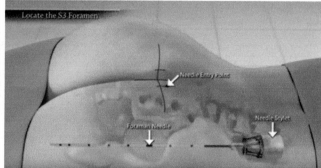

Figure 31.3   Sacral nerve stimulation (SNS).

There are seven different programs on the device. If the patient is not doing well on one program, another one can be selected. The intensity, which controls the strength of the stimulator, can be adjusted as well. Initially, it is turned on with 0 intensity and then increased by 0.1 every few seconds until the child feels a flutter in the bicycle seat. This feeling will naturally subside in 1–5 days. This does not mean that the SNS has stopped working. It is just an indicator that the patient has adapted to the device.

Patients may complain of pain radiating down the leg. To evaluate if the pain is related to the SNS, you can turn the device off for 3 days. If there is no further pain while the device is off and then the pain returns when the device is on, then it is related to the stimulator. Changing the program is the first step to eliminate the radiating pain. Then the intensity is set again. If the pain continues, then most likely a change in the pulse wave setting is needed. This setting controls how far from the sacral space the stimulation or signals occur. This parameter can only be adjusted by the company representative or the care provider under the representative's guidance. Changing the parameter settings cannot be done remotely. Often, with this slight change, the radiating pain can be resolved.

RECOMMENDED READING

Sulkowski JP, Nacion KM, Deans KJ, Minneci PC, Levitt MA, Mousa HM, Alpert SA, Teich S. Sacral nerve stimulation: A promising therapy for fecal and urinary incontinence and constipation in children. *J Pediatr Surg.* 2015 Oct; 50(10): 1644–1647.

Vriesman MH, Wang L, Park C, Diefenbach KA, Levitt MA, Wood RJ, Alpert SA, Benninga MA, Vaz K, Yacob D, Di Lorenzo C, Lu PL. Comparison of antegrade continence enema treatment and sacral nerve stimulation for children with severe functional constipation and fecal incontinence. *Neurogastroenterol Motil.* 2020 Aug; 32(8): e13809.

DECOMPRESSION VENT FOR CHRONIC INTESTINAL PSEUDO-OBSTRUCTION (CIPO)

Hollow visceral myopathy is a fatal variant of chronic intestinal pseudo-obstruction (CIPO) that leads to progressive dilatation of the gastrointestinal tract which usually starts from the colon and progresses proximally. The disease has no known cure, and all interventions are palliative. Life expectancy is only up to the second

> No matter how you squash and squeeze, it has to fit one disease.
>
> **– Fred Ryckman**

decade of life. Placing a low-profile gastrostomy tube in the splenic flexure of the colon using a colonoscope, in the same manner in which one would insert a PEG tube, allows for patients to intermittently vent air, decreasing the massive distension that occurs from being unable to pass flatus (Figure 31.4). Placement of the tube can be assisted with the help of laparoscopy which offers direct visualization and assurance that other gastrointestinal tract structures are not injured in the process.

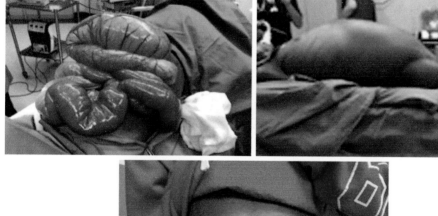

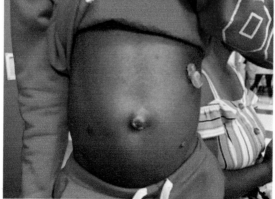

Figure 31.4   Decompression vent for CIPO.

RECOMMENDED READING

Pironi L, Sasdelli AS. Management of the patient with chronic intestinal pseudo-obstruction and intestinal failure. *Gastroenterol Clin North Am.* 2019 Dec; 48(4): 513–524.

IDIOPATHIC RECTAL PROLAPSE

A 7-year-old female comes to your clinic with daily rectal prolapse, shown in Figure 31.5.

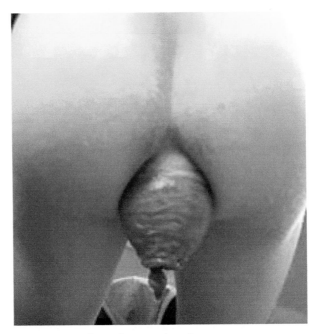

Figure 31.5 Idiopathic rectal prolapse.

What is your routine evaluation for such a patient? What testing is needed?

To evaluate "idiopathic prolapse," the most common cause is constipation, which needs to be treated, but also consider cystic fibrosis, malnutrition, a spinal anomaly, and any condition causing hypermotility. Endoscopy is vital to be sure it is not a polyp that is prolapsing or inflamed mucosa representing underlying inflammatory bowel disease.

If you decide this patient needs surgery, what would be your intervention?

If, after ruling out all of the above and treating constipation, the prolapse continues, then you will need to intervene surgically. A transanal Swenson to remove the distal 6–8 cm of the rectum works well. Sclerosing agents (hpertonic saline) and laparoscopic rectopexy are other options.

FIFTEEN-YEAR-OLD FEMALE WITH ABDOMINAL PAIN AND AMENORRHEA

A 15-year-old female presents for evaluation with abdominal pain and amenorrhea. The patient has a normal urethra and normal anus. Her MRI is shown in Figure 31.6.

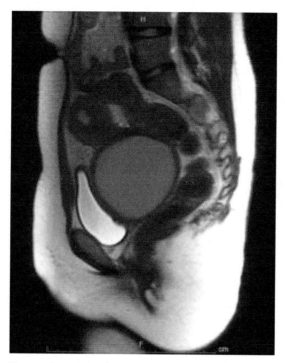

Figure 31.6 MRI showing hematometrcolpos.

What is the diagnosis?

There is a massive hematometrocolpos visualized on the MRI (presumably with retained blood from menses). Given the age and history of the patient (amenorrhea at 15 years), the differential diagnosis includes an imperforate hymen, a transverse vaginal septum, or a distal vaginal atresia.

What treatment would you choose? When would you intervene?

Urgent treatment should be first directed at draining the hydrocolpos and relieving the pain. Next, to establish the diagnosis, the patient should undergo an EUA and vaginoscopy. It is very important to measure the hormones to be sure that the ovaries are functional. If not, the patient may need hormonal manipulation. Then, elective surgery for definitive repair can be planned.

An imperforate hymen can be incised. A longitudinal vaginal septum can be surgically removed. A transverse vaginal septum can be managed by incision and marsupialization. If vaginoplasty is needed, a vaginal pull-through is a good option since the vagina is very dilated.

If a laparoscopic mobilization of the distal vagina does not reach, there are several options for vaginal replacement (buccal mucosa and OASIS™ matrix graft can be used to make a neovagina). If she is not amenable to surgery now, the dilated vagina must be drained (can be done percutaneously), and then she would require hormonal suppression.

POSTERIOR SAGITTAL ANORECTOPLASTY IN A PATIENT WITH CAUDAL DUPLICATION SYNDROME

A 6-year-old male with caudal duplication syndrome (CDS) presented to clinic with a persistent fistula between his right ureter and colon (Figure 31.7).

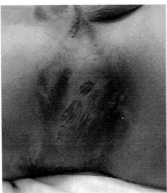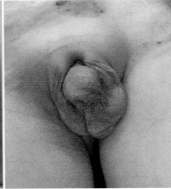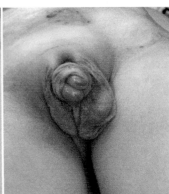

Figure 31.7   Caudal duplication syndrome.

There are those that don't know, and those that don't know that they don't know.

– Contributed by: Marc Levitt

CDS is a rare syndrome wherein the structures derived from the embryonic cloaca and notochord are duplicated to various degrees. This patient had a duplicated colon, rectum, bladder, penis, and urethra for which he had undergone multiple surgeries at an outside institution. He ultimately had a megacolon with diverting colostomy created at age 1 which was complicated by a rectourethral fistula. The fistula was taken down at age 4. After his colostomy was reversed, he developed a recurrent fistula. Therefore, a diverting ileostomy was created, and the fistula was repaired with a left thigh soft tissue interposition. Despite this repair, he developed a fistula between his right urethra and the megacolon suture line and presented for evaluation. With the diverting ileostomy in place, he was no longer having any output from his rectums. He was, however, having urinary incontinence along with recurrent UTIs.

On evaluation, he was found to have a well-developed anus on the left, connected to his rectums. He had functioning sphincter muscles on the right but no true anus. In between the two, there was scar and fat tissue from his prior lipomyelomeningocele resection. Owing to the variability of malformations found within CDS, it is important to consider each patient individually and form a surgical plan in a multidisciplinary approach. In this case, a collaboration with urology proceeded.

The anal canal on the patient's left was preserved. The rectum was mobilized, and a rectoplasty was performed to connect the duplicated rectums and create one lumen. The skin from the island of tissue in the center was removed, and the fat was preserved to cover the fistula repair. In conjunction with urology performing an intraoperative cystoscopy, the fistula was identified between the right rectum and right bladder neck and was subsequently taken down and oversewn. With the island of tissue removed and utilized to bolster the fistula repair, the right and left sphincters could now be mobilized and joined together around the preserved anus to create one rectum and anus (Figure 31.8).

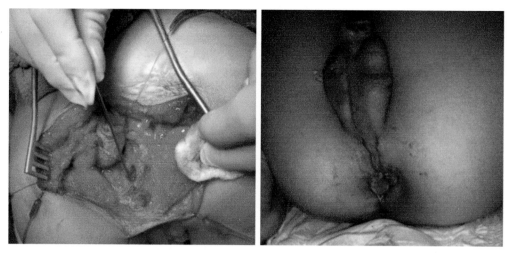

Figure 31.8 Left picture shows a fistula probe in the rectourethral fistula. The right picture shows the final result of the anoplasty.

RECOMMENDED READING

Samuk I, Levitt M, Dlugy E, Kravarusic D, Ben-Meir D, Rajz G, Konen O, Freud E. Caudal duplication syndrome: The vital role of a multidisciplinary approach and staged correction. *Eur J Pediatr Surg Rep.* 2016 Dec; 4(1): 1–5.

INDEX

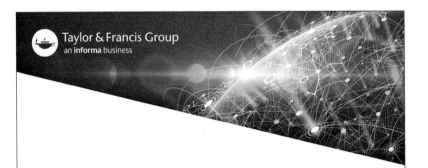